PENGUIN BOOKS

LISTEN TO YOUR PAIN

Dr. Ben E. Benjamin—educator, author, and therapist to people suffering from pain and stress-related problems—earned his Ph.D. in sports medicine and education. He has been in private practice for more than twenty years and is presently practicing in Boston and New York City. He developed the profession of muscular therapy and has written two previous books on his work: *Are You Tense?: The Benjamin System of Muscular Therapy*, on the theory and techniques of muscular therapy, and *Sports Without Pain*, a comprehensive system of exercises for the prevention of injuries. In 1975 he founded the Muscular Therapy Institute, a unique three-year program that accents personal and professional development as well as professional skills. Additionally, as part of his work, he developed a form of communications-skills training that is useful in reducing stress and its manifestations in the body. Dr. Benjamin has taught workshops and courses at several hospitals and many universities throughout the country and has dedicated his life to investigating new ways to help in the treatment of pain, injury, and stress.

Listen to Your Pain

The Active Person's Guide to Understanding,
Identifying, and Treating Pain and Injury

BEN E. BENJAMIN, Ph.D.
with Gale Borden, M.D.

Illustrations by Norman Campbell

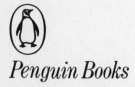

Penguin Books

PENGUIN BOOKS
Published by the Penguin Group
Penguin Books USA Inc.,
375 Hudson Street, New York, New York 10014, U.S.A.
Penguin Books Ltd, 27 Wrights Lane, London W8 5TZ, England
Penguin Books Australia Ltd, Ringwood, Victoria, Australia
Penguin Books Canada Ltd, 10 Alcorn Avenue,
Toronto, Ontario, Canada M4V 3B2
Penguin Books (N.Z.) Ltd, 182–190 Wairau Road, Auckland 10, New Zealand

Penguin Books Ltd, Registered Offices:
Harmondsworth, Middlesex, England

First published in the United States of America
in simultaneous hardcover and paperback editions by
Viking Penguin Inc. 1984

20   19   18

ISBN 0 14 00.6687 X

Printed in the United States of America

Set in Linotron Century Expanded
Designed by Ann Gold

Photographs on pages 300–301 courtesy J. Peter Happel
Copyright © J. Peter Happel, 1984

To Dr. Elsworth F. Baker
Whose humility and decency have taught me so much

To Dr. Milne Ongley and Dr. James Cyriax
Who gave me the knowledge to understand pain and injury

And to Lea Delacour
My deep and true friend for many years

Acknowledgments

Along the way to publication, many people have helped me, and I wish to recognize and thank them: Perry White, Ara Fitzgerald, Gail Stevens, and Roberta Folkedahl for their assistance in preparing the first draft; special thanks to Carol Hess for help in polishing the second draft and for endless retyping of the manuscript. To Jim Robinson my thanks for his astute criticisms and tireless assistance.

I am grateful for the advice of Dr. David Jones and Dr. Lynn Anderson, who helped me simplify the chapters on the neck and back. I am also indebted to Dr. James Cyriax, who through his teaching seminars gave me much important information for which I had been searching for ten years. Amanda Vaill, my enthusiastic and supportive editor, has my appreciation for her patience and suggestions. My deepest gratitude goes to Dr. Milne Ongley, who shared with me his vast knowledge of orthopedic medicine and taught me some of the most important things I've ever learned.

The sensitive and elegant illustrations by Norman Campbell were diligently worked and reworked to meet both of our critical satisfactions. It was a pleasure to work with him and see him translate anatomy to art. I thank him.

My thanks to Fran Salkin for assisting me in the rewriting of the final draft; her ingenuity, superb writing skills, and hard work have added touches of humor and clarity. Her persistent and critical honesty and creative imagination helped me make what could have been a boring treatise into what I hope will be not only a useful but an enjoyable book.

—Ben E. Benjamin, Ph.D.
New York, New York
Lincoln, Massachusetts

Author's Note

Knowledge is an ever-changing process, nowhere more so than in Western medicine, where information we believe to be true today may prove to be incomplete or false tomorrow. In a science less than a hundred years old, there is much learning that is still trial and error; sometimes doctors successfully treat an illness or injury but do not know why the treatment works.

New treatments are constantly evolving. This book on pain and injury would have to encompass volumes if it were to include all injuries and all treatments. So I have selected the injuries most common among active people and have included all the treatments I am personally familiar with. For example, I have left out ultrasound and acupuncture because I am not familiar with their effectiveness. I am also excluding several treatments that are successfully used in Europe because they are still illegal in the United States. In this book you may find suggested treatments that you aren't familiar with, e.g., deep frictioning and the use of proliferants. These are very effective treatments which are gaining in popularity in the United States.

At various points throughout this book, I have referred to an earlier book of mine, *Sports Without Pain*. This book is currently unavailable in bookstores but can be ordered from Relaxation Tools, Inc., P.O. Box 1045, New York, N.Y. 10025.

In writing this book I had invaluable help from Dr. Gale Borden on a number of sections. He advised me on all the technical medical aspects and wrote the Appendix, the section for doctors. In addition, he critically reviewed the entire manuscript and was available for consultation. He joins with me in hoping this book will help you broaden your base of understanding about pain and injury so that you may choose more intelligently from your options of treatment and care.

Contents

PART II

PART III

Glossary

Here is a list of common medical terms that will come up again and again in the discussion of injuries. Because they're so often misunderstood, I've defined them to eliminate confusion. I have tried to keep more technical terms to a minimum; where they must be used, they're defined as they come up.

ANTERIOR   Anatomical structures that lie toward the front of the body.

ARTHRITIS   A shrinking and stiffening of the fibers within a joint. There are twelve types of arthritis.

BURSA   A fluid-filled sac that cushions movement, for example, as tendons slide over bones.

CALCIFY   To harden. Liquid calcium turns to solid matter.

CORTICOSTEROID   The umbrella term for all anti-inflammatory steroid drugs, e.g., hydrocortisone, prednisone, triamcinolone, and others.

DISC   Spongy cartilage material that cushions and separates the vertebrae.

FRACTURE   A crack or break of a bone.

HEMATOMA   A crush injury where many small blood vessels are broken. Blood seeps into the surrounding tissue and a bruise and/or lump appears.

INFLAMMATION   Irritation, swelling, reddening, and heat combined.

JOINT   Where any two bones meet.

LATERAL   Anatomical structures that lie toward the right or left side of the body.

LIGAMENT   Tough, fibrous tissue that connects bone to bone.

MEDIAL   Anatomical structures that lie toward the middle of the body.

PERIOSTEUM   The membranelike structure that covers all bones; it can be thought of as a bone skin.

POSTERIOR   Anatomical structures that lie toward the back of the body.

RUPTURE   Complete tearing apart of a muscle, tendon, or ligament.

SPRAIN OR STRAIN   An irritation, slight swelling, or microscopic tearing of tendons, muscles, or ligaments. Usually strain refers to tendons or muscles, and sprain refers to ligaments, but it is common for them to be used interchangeably.

TEAR   A major or minor separation of muscle, tendon, or ligament fiber. We use the word primarily to refer to minor microscopic tears.

TENDINITIS   An irritated, swollen, strained tendon.

TENDON   Tough, fibrous tissue that connects muscle to bone.

I.

Introduction

Listening to your pain isn't easy—even when it shouts. The language is foreign, and though there are many signs and signals, they make no sense without a guide to interpret them. If you are reading this you have probably had, or are currently suffering from, a pain or injury that frustrated, inconvenienced, or bewildered you.

Pain can be a lonely experience. It imprisons you, locking you away from your physical pleasures. If the pain continues over time, depression can begin to intrude destructively into your daily activities. Often your isolation increases as you struggle through a maze of confusing, conflicting professional opinions, expectations, and disappointments.

At the age of fourteen, I had a serious and debilitating back injury and began a seemingly endless search for help. My pain was so severe that even simple acts such as getting out of bed and walking were extremely difficult, and after a year of trying many doctors I finally found someone who could help me. This painful ordeal stimulated my interest in understanding and solving pain problems.

There are many injuries that are easily diagnosed and successfully treated; however, pain and injury are in general rather poorly understood aspects of medicine. The causes are often elusive, the diagnosis is frequently mistaken, and, as a consequence, treatments fail. In part, the root of this problem has been that existing knowledge of injuries has not been drawn together in a concise form.

3

Where are the answers? I hope you will find many of them right here. This book is designed to answer your unheard questions. It gives you the knowledge to understand the many signals your body sends out when you are injured and helps you learn how to communicate these to your doctor. *Listen to Your Pain* tells you what it is, how you got it, how to evaluate it, and what your treatment choices are. It takes highly technical material and presents it in a way that is easily understood.

This is a book for people in pain, whether from an athletic injury, an accident, or from slow wear and tear; it's for anyone who wants to understand the injury process.

Throughout the text we emphasize that certain types of injuries need immediate medical attention; all injuries involving paralysis or broken bones require a physician's care and therefore are not covered in this book. If you have a sudden severe pain or obvious swelling anywhere, see a doctor before referring to this text. Fortunately, most injuries are not so serious. Strains, sprains, and inflammations that we talk about throughout this book account for 90 percent of the most common athletic and everyday living injuries. However, if you are in any doubt about the seriousness of your injury, see your doctor.

There are four steps to follow in using this book effectively.

1. Thoroughly read Part I to gain the background information you will need to understand your injuries and the treatment choices available.
2. Turn to the section in Part II on the area of the body you have injured. At the beginning of each section you will find material that will help you determine and understand which injury you might have.
3. Now turn to the section that discusses your particular injury. Here you will find how to evaluate and treat it.
4. Part III contains chapters on Rehabilitation, Reconditioning, and Prevention. Here you will find specific exercises that can help you get well.

The final section of this book is not for you; it's a mini-manual for your doctor on injection techniques he may not be familiar with.

Following this procedure carefully, you will be more informed and less confused about your injury and the pain it is causing you. Complex material is presented along with hundreds of drawings so that it can be readily understood by individuals without medical training. I hope this book will help you attain—and then maintain—your good physical health.

1

Pain and What It Tells You

Pain is a signal that something is wrong. If it is mild and disappears quickly it's probably nothing to worry about. However, if the pain is severe, or persists for over a week, your body is trying to tell you something. Take it seriously! Catching an injury early always makes it easier to take care of. There are many people who fail to listen to their body's early warning signals, and as a result they have compounded their injuries, crippling themselves with unnecessary pain for months and even years.

Pain comes in many forms. It can be mildly annoying or excruciating. It can be sharply piercing, it can be a dull ache, or it can tingle or burn. The cause of your pain might be a torn ligament or tendon, a pinched or bruised nerve, a broken or diseased bone, or even an emotional or psychological problem.

There are many times when pain is your signal that you should see a physician. However, when to see your doctor is not a black-and-white issue. It will always be a matter of judgment, but here are some guidelines to help you make that decision. See your doctor

1. if your pain is severe;
2. if there is swelling;
3. if you hear any cracking or snapping sounds at the moment of injury;
4. if you cannot perform normal activities;
5. if there is nausea, dizziness, blurred vision, paralysis, weakness or disturbed excretory functioning following an accident or injury;
6. if your pain continues beyond seven to ten days.

In certain parts of the body pain can be deceiving. It is possible to have an injury in one part of the body and feel pain somewhere else. For example, you might have a pinched nerve in your lower back and feel the pain only in your calf. This phenomenon is known as *referred pain*.

Referred Pain

HOW WE PERCEIVE PAIN
The brain is our interpreter of pain. The surface of the brain, the cerebral cortex, is where the sensations felt in the body are translated into the message, *pain*. But before reaching the cerebral cortex the pain has passed through several pathways that can alter our perception of the location of the pain.

If you prick your finger, sensory nerves in your finger lose no time in transmitting this pain to the corresponding point on the cortex as a direct message. But the brain surface is not the only perceiver of pain. Depending upon what you've injured and its location, pathways for pain perception may be intercepted in the spinal cord. Sensation may also be sidetracked in the thalamus, the centrally located pain center, before going on to the cortex. A pinched nerve in your lower back is a good example of how referred pain works. Pressure on one nerve can be felt as lower-back pain, thigh pain, or a very specific ache in your big toe.

DERMATOMES

When pain is referred it follows specific patterns based on embryological development. The human embryo develops out of thirty-two original segments. Each segment—or *dermatome*—will eventually become a certain area of the body. Understanding and distinguishing dermatomes can be confusing because many of the developing segments are not connected and continuous. For example, one dermatome (C8) in the neck will include one neck vertebra with the surrounding ligaments and nerves, the lower portion of the forearm, half the palm, and the outer three fingers. Thus an injury in your neck can be felt as a pain in your hand. Even in continuous dermatomes (C5), such as the one containing the shoulder, upper arm, and forearm, a

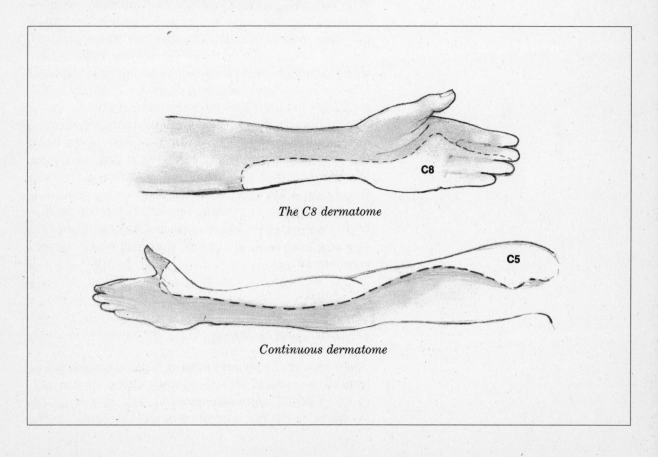

The C8 dermatome

Continuous dermatome

specific injury can be felt anywhere along that dermatome. In many cases the pain is *not felt at all* in the injured
area but is referred to another part of the dermatome. We
have known about dermatomes for a long time, but the
part they play in the phenomenon of referred pain had not
been explored until two physicians from England, Lewis
and Kellgren, rediscovered their usefulness in diagnosing
injuries in the 1930s and 1940s.

It's important to keep in mind, when evaluating neck,
shoulder, and lower-back injuries, that the pain from
these injuries will often be felt in a distant part of the dermatome. These are the major areas that commonly refer
pain. Injuries to the elbow, knee, thigh, calf, and ankle are
easier to evaluate and understand because there is very
little referred pain in these places. Familiarity with referred pain patterns makes diagnosing your injury easier,
but since most people do not understand these patterns,
referred pain usually confuses them. Who would believe
that a pain in the hand is caused by an injury in the neck?
Many people, when given their diagnosis, suddenly lose all
confidence in their physician's professional skill.

In addition to the problem of referred pain, there is also
difficulty in accurately perceiving pain deep in the body.
Our brains can more readily perceive the location of pains
caused by injuries that are near the surface of the skin.
When pain is felt deep inside the body, as in a joint, it is
more difficult for our minds to pinpoint its location precisely. In these cases we feel the pain in a wider and more diffuse area, and so we are unsure of exactly where our pain
is coming from.

Psychogenic Pain

When pain is elusive and evades diagnosis, some physicians, from a lack of experience, may categorize it as psychogenic pain. Their assumption is that the pain you're
experiencing has no physical cause and therefore must be

emotional in origin. At times you're given the sense that you're making up or exaggerating your discomfort, when in fact your injury just cannot be found. While there *is* psychogenic pain that is entirely emotionally based, and that can only be treated by treating the emotional cause, certain strange and uncommon neck and back injuries, especially postsurgical pain, often defy diagnosis by even the most experienced physicians.

One type of elusive pain can be caused by long-standing (chronic) muscle tension. Another form of elusive pain comes from a sudden rise in muscle tension. Both of these are often triggered by increased life pressures which add an overload of emotional stress to the nervous system. In discomfort owing to muscle tension there is usually no torn muscle fiber, although real pain is felt. The discomfort from emotionally caused muscle tension can be experienced in a generalized area or can be sharp and piercing, as in the pain of a headache.

Points to remember: Every pain has a cause. If you find it and treat it properly you will get better. If injections, massage, surgery, or other forms of treatment are applied to the general area but miss the exact location of the injury, you will not get better. It is not enough that the diagnosis is generally right. It must be exact in order for you to recover. In cases of severe continuing pain, always see a doctor. Only a physician can screen out the possibility that your pain is coming from a serious injury or disease. What you interpret as an arm pain could actually be a heart attack.

2

Basic Structures of the Body and What Happens When You Injure Them

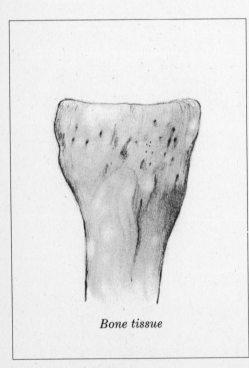

Bone tissue

What happens to the various parts of our bodies when they are injured? What makes the injury remain painful for months? Tendon or ligament fibers tear apart like a rope that has frayed. Other commonly injured structures, such as bones, bursas, and discs, also have characteristic forms of injury, and understanding these will lead to more intelligent and productive treatment choices. This chapter will discuss the parts of our bodies that are most susceptible to injury and what actually happens to them when they are injured.

Bones

Our bones give our body structure and form. They are covered by a skinlike material called "periosteum." Under this periosteal covering there is a fluid that bathes and nourishes the bones. Injuries to the bone occur in varying degrees. A break is a complete severing of bone. A greenstick fracture is a cracking of the bone. A stress fracture (often referred to as a fatigue fracture) is a very small fracture (or crack) in a bone that occurs over a period of time, usually through rhythmic and repeated stress (e.g., from running).

Bones usually heal fairly well; in fact, healed fractures often leave the bone stronger than it was before the injury. It's as though you have added a coating of super-glue around the bone. Stress fractures of small bones usually take six to eight weeks to heal; other fractures may take between two and twelve months to heal, depending on the bone and where it's fractured. If a fracture is not properly diagnosed and treated, it can heal in a poor position and create ongoing problems.

Bone pain is not always caused by fractures. You can bruise a bone by banging into something or by a repeated pounding motion. The resulting condition is called periostitis (*peri*, from the periosteum "boneskin"; *ostitis*, meaning inflammation of the bone), in which the bone covering swells with extra fluid to protect and heal the bruised bone beneath it.

Bone spurs are another source of pain. A spur is an abnormal bone growth that creates a spurlike bump on the bone. If a spur occurs in the foot and is painful, it may have to be removed. However, there are nonpainful spurs; for example, if there is a spur at the outside of the knee, it may be aesthetically unappealing, but it may be harmless and not need to be removed.

Cartilage

Cartilage is a flexible and compressible structure that takes many different forms in the body.

It forms certain flexible structures, such as our nose and ears; we have special cartilages in our knees, called *menisci*, and others in our back, called *discs*. At joints, the ends of our bones are covered with a special type of cartilage that looks and feels something like Teflon; it allows the bones to glide over one another without rubbing each other away.

Cartilage has almost no blood vessels and almost no

nerves, so that when it cracks or breaks it rarely heals. It also rarely hurts. When we tear or crack the shock-absorbing cartilage in our knee or in our back, the pain we feel is not actually from the torn cartilage itself. What causes pain is that the cartilage moves into the wrong place, and either presses on a vital structure, such as a nerve, or causes unnatural tensions on ligaments, thus producing pain.

DISCS

With the exception of the first two vertebrae in your neck, each vertebra in your spine is separated from its neighbors by cushioning pieces of cartilage called *discs*. A great deal of pain and suffering is caused by disc problems. For example, if you've suffered from a back spasm, a loss of strength in your arm, pain and burning, tingling, or numbness down your leg, you may have had a major or minor disc problem. Neck pain, center- and lower-back pain, and pain down the leg, often called sciatic pain, are easily comprehensible once the relationship between discs and nerves is understood.

The cushioning discs are circular and made up of two different types of cartilage. Their outer rim is a dense fibrous material which is somewhat flexible. The inner cartilage of the disc is soft and squishy, like very thick jelly. This substance functions hydraulically to cushion against jarring movements such as walking, jumping, and running. Over the years, the soft central portion of the disc can harden into a tough, calcified (solid) cartilage. This hardening process is complete by age sixty in some people. This is a natural consequence of aging, and causes the spine to be more brittle, less resilient to shocks.

Discs can cause trouble in two ways: the disc can crack, causing a piece of the hard rim to chip off and lodge itself next to a nerve (A), which results in pain. Or the outer hard, fibrous tissue cracks and the soft inner portion of the disc—the nucleus pulposus—slowly oozes out until it presses on a nerve or some other sensitive structure, causing pain. Since this inner substance is now out of its natu-

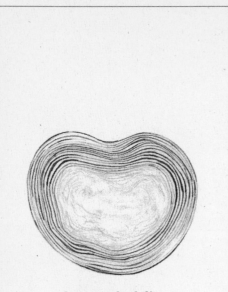

Intervertebral disc

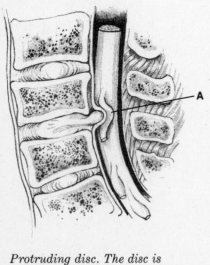

Protruding disc. The disc is pressing on a nerve (A), which causes pain.

ral environment, it receives no nourishment and in some cases shrivels up and is absorbed by the body. However, you remain in discomfort until this process is completed, which can take a year or longer.

Disc problems cause many pains in the neck and shoulder as well as the most serious lower-back disabilities, sometimes requiring surgery. Many of the symptoms and much of the pain they cause can be mimicked by torn and sprained ligaments, leading to tremendous confusion in diagnosis.

Scar Tissue

The fibers of a tendon, a muscle, or a ligament are like the strings of a violin, in that they run parallel to one another. When fibers tear, it is as though the strings were cut. Ideally, the fibers should heal parallel again (like getting new violin strings), but often this doesn't happen. Instead, in the body's enthusiasm to heal, the fibers not only join end to end, but they also stick to those running parallel to them, as if all of your violin strings were glued together. When they are stressed through use, the strings or the fibers retear and the area becomes painful and inflamed. As the fibers heal again, they stick and mat together in all directions, forming internal scar tissue. This is painful, rigid tissue which creates chronic muscle, tendon, or ligament injuries. Painful scar tissue occurs more frequently in tendons and ligaments than in muscles.

Muscles

Muscles control movement by contracting and shortening. This is the only action they can perform. Muscles are red because they are filled with many blood vessels which supply them with oxygen and food and remove carbon dioxide and waste products. They heal very quickly because they have so much blood circulating within them. Muscles have thousands of separate fibers which run *in the same direction as the movement they perform*. For instance, the bi-

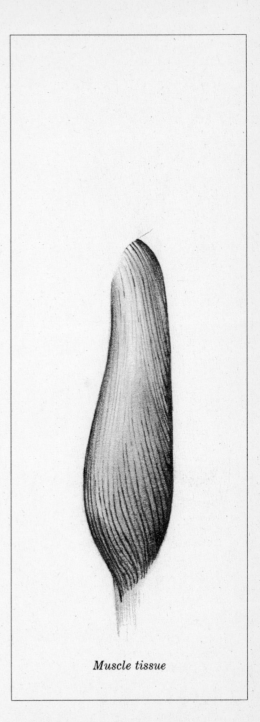

Muscle tissue

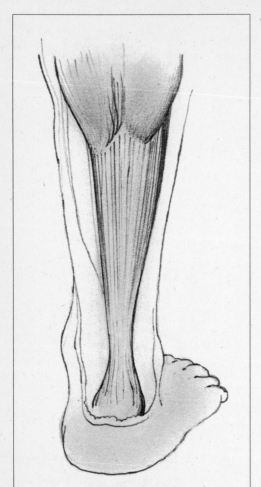

Achilles tendon

ceps muscle in your upper arm has fibers that run up and down the arm; they enable you to bend and straighten your arm in that direction. Other muscles in your chest and shoulder have fibers running horizontally, and these muscles enable you to move your arm from side to side. When you injure a muscle, it hurts to move it.

Muscles can be injured in three ways: muscle fibers may be strained slightly by excessive activity and swell. This swelling usually causes a mild pain over a wide area which disappears in a few days. A more serious muscle injury occurs when a small group of muscle fibers tears apart. This is referred to as a muscle-belly tear. When a small number of fibers tear the healing is fairly rapid, usually taking a week or two. The more muscle fibers torn, the more severe the injury, causing greater pain and longer healing time. The third type of muscle injury is a hematoma. When a muscle experiences a severe fall or blow, and a crushing injury occurs, many of the blood vessels break, allowing the blood to seep out into a broad area.

Tendons

A tendon is made up of tough, fibrous, ropelike material which is smooth, white, and usually flat and shiny. It acts as a connecting link between muscles and bones. Tendons will not stretch, except microscopically, and they do not contract as muscles do. They merely link muscles to bones. Tendons have very little blood supply and can take a long, long time to heal after an injury.

Tendons are one of the most commonly injured structures in the body. When a tendon is injured, only some of its fibers actually tear; it rarely rips completely in half. What happens is that some fibers, say fifty out of ten thousand, tear in a given tendon. The higher the proportion of fibers torn, the more severe the tear and the pain. For you to feel better, the torn structure must heal, and it must heal correctly and fully. When healing is incomplete, you remain vulnerable to reinjury because the tendon is now structurally weak. If tendon injuries do not receive proper treatment, they can take months or even years to heal.

Many people assume they have injured a muscle when in fact they have injured a tendon. It's hard to know the difference without a thorough knowledge of anatomy because tendons and muscles are attached to each other and function as one unit. The easiest way to tell whether you've injured a muscle or a tendon is to compare the location of your pain with the anatomical diagrams you will find later on in this book.

Injuries to the tendon occur in one of three places (see illustration):

1. The tendon can tear away slightly from where it is attached to the bone. This is a very frequent place of injury.
2. Some of the fibers in the main body of the tendon tear.
3. The tendon tears where it attaches to the muscle.

TENDINITIS

Tendinitis means the tendon is partially torn, as in 1, 2, and 3 above. Inflamed or torn tendons take a long time to heal because they do not have a large blood supply, and when the tendon is restressed it frequently retears. It often heals badly, with a lot of scar tissue, and tends to be restrained again and again as described in Scar Tissue, above.

TENOSYNOVITIS

Tenosynovitis is another type of tendon injury. Certain tendons are surrounded by a sheath containing a fluid—called synovial fluid—that bathes and nourishes them. When the tendon moves, the sheath remains stationary as the tendon glides within it, as a piston moves within a lubricated shaft. If the internal surface of the tendon becomes irritated and roughened, pain is caused when the tendon and the sheath rub against each other in normal movement. There is often a detectable grinding or crack-

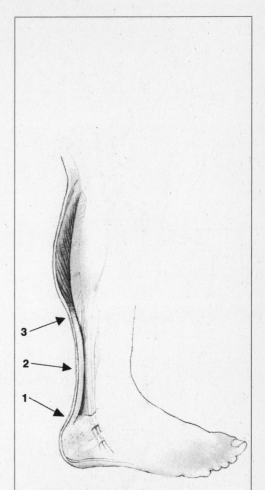

Injuries to the tendon may occur in one of these three places.

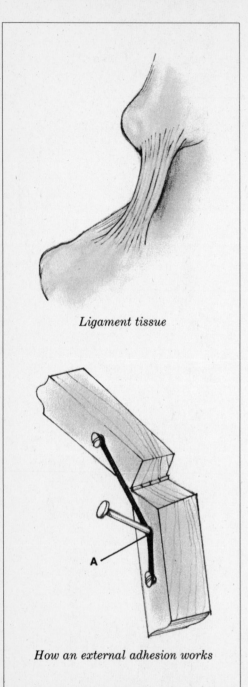

Ligament tissue

How an external adhesion works

ling sound heard at the tendon. This can be a very stubborn injury.

INFLAMED TENDONS

Inflamed tendons without tears are a less serious type of tendon injury. A minor overexertion or trauma can cause a slight swelling (inflammation) of some of the individual fibers, creating internal pressures and slight pain. This type of injury is usually self-healing with a week to ten days of rest.

Ligaments

A ligament is a tough, fibrous piece of material which looks white and ropy and has a very limited blood supply. Its structure is similar to that of a tendon but its purpose is different. The function of ligaments is to limit range of motion and to hold all your bones together. Several ligaments hold the thigh bone to the shin bone and the lower leg to the ankle; others hold the bones of your spine together.

Ligaments are not supposed to stretch, except microscopically.* If we do stretch them, either through an accident or through poor stretching exercises, we cause the joint they support to become permanently weak and unstable.

Ligaments can be damaged quite easily, especially in the knee and ankle. When a ligament is injured it can tear partially or completely in two, often needing surgical repair. What generally happens is that some of the ligament fiber tears slightly, like the fraying of a rope. When even a slight tear occurs, the body's inflammation process starts quickly and things begin to heal, although often erratically. Many times the fibers heal together poorly, as described in the violin example on page 13, and become matted, so that when you put stress on the ligament again with activity it retears.

*Five ligaments, called yellow ligaments, *can* stretch.

Owing to their poor blood supply, ligaments heal slowly and often poorly. And sometimes, as the fibers of the ligament begin to heal, they adhere to the bone (A *opposite, below*) near it with external scar tissue. Then the underlying bone cannot move freely, as it was intended to do. This is called an *adhesion*. When this occurs, the fibers retear after moderate exertion, this time pulling away from the bone they weren't supposed to be attached to. The repeated cycle of adhering and tearing is why ligament injuries to the knee often become long-standing.

Bursas

A bursa (A) is a fluid-filled sac that usually lies between a tendon and a bone, though in some places it lies between a ligament and a bone. You have a bursa in the shoulder which lies between the shoulder tendons and the bone of the shoulder (see point A in the illustration). It acts as padding and allows the tendon to glide under the bone without becoming irritated or torn. Without the bursa, the tendon would rub directly over bone and slowly wear away. An irritated bursa can produce pain that lasts for years if not properly treated. This is called *bursitis*. What happens is that the bursa becomes too full of fluid and causes pain as the bone moves and the tendon rides over the bursa. In some cases, a painful scar forms within the bursa, causing pain on movement. Even though we don't know what causes bursitis, it can be treated effectively.

Fascia

Fascia is a peculiar and extremely varied tissue: in some areas it is as thick and strong as a ligament; in others it is as thin and fragile as tissue paper. Its primary function is to cover, protect, and separate all of the muscles of the body. Every muscle is wrapped separately in this tissue-like fascia, which enables the muscles to slide easily on one another. In several places, the fascia serves the function of

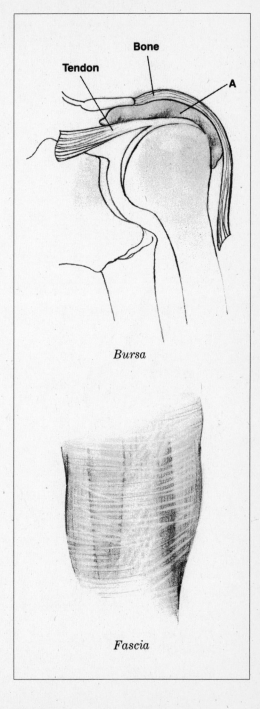

Bursa

Fascia

a ligament or tendon; and the fascia in these places get injured the same way ligaments and tendons do.

Running injuries often involve fascia. One that we see all the time is a nasty ubiquitous pain on the bottom of the foot, especially toward the heel, that visits runners when they first stand up in the morning, vanishing mysteriously after a few minutes of walking, only to return at the end of a long run.

Joints

Joints are usually difficult to visualize. A joint is simply where any two bones meet. Everybody knows you have a

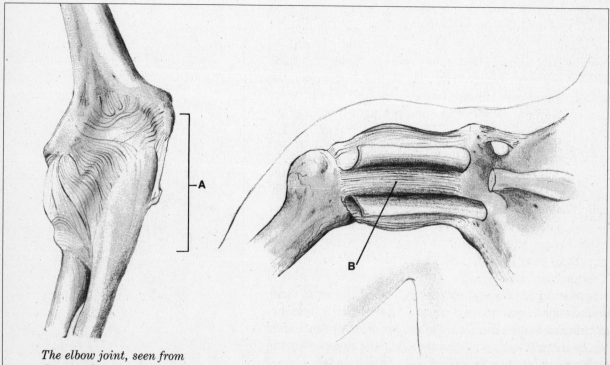

The elbow joint, seen from the outside

Shoulder joint—interior view

knee joint, but between each of your vertebrae there is also a joint, and even your little finger has three joints.

Joints that move primarily in two directions are called hinge joints—the ankle and wrist, for example, are hinge joints. Others—like the shoulder and hip, which move in any direction—are called ball-and-socket joints.

Every joint is surrounded and encased in a "joint capsule" (A on opposite page). This is an air-tight covering made of the same thick ropelike material that forms ligaments. The joint capsule protects the joint and contains a fluid called synovial fluid, which lubricates and nourishes the joint. The inner surface of the joint capsule (B) is lined with a thin, sensitive membrane called the synovial membrane. This membrane produces the synovial fluid.

When a joint is injured and painful it is because the synovial membrane and/or the joint capsule are irritated and inflamed. In some cases the joint swells with excess fluid to prevent movement that would cause further damage; in others the walls of the joint capsule shrink and stiffen, causing barriers to movement.

LOOSE BODY

A mysterious phenomenon that occurs in joints and is frequently missed in diagnosis is called a "loose body." This term refers to a chipped piece of bone or cartilage floating inside a joint. When this piece of loose bone or cartilage (A) is dislodged it can cause severe pain. The piece continually floats around in the joint, but sometimes it becomes lodged in a position that prevents the full movement of the joint. Frequently a knee gets stuck—if you're lucky, you can shake your leg and jiggle the chip into a quiet corner. This problem also occurs in the hip, and the elbow, and less often in the ankle. People who have a "loose body" describe walking along quite normally, then suddenly experiencing a severe, sharp pain for no apparent reason. They shake the affected joint, the pain usually goes away, and they resume their walk.

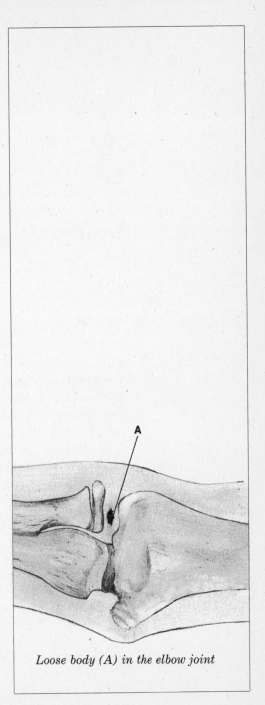

Loose body (A) in the elbow joint

3

Causes of Injury

There are thousands of people who used to love running but sadly found that over the years their knees began to hurt so badly that they were forced to abandon their source of pleasure. Many avid tennis players have experienced similar problems from slow damage to their elbows and shoulders. In both running and tennis, as in other sports, certain parts of the body are particularly vulnerable to injury.* If you understand the causes of injuries, you have a good chance of preventing the injuries from happening. With adequate knowledge, injuries common to tennis, running, skiing, and so forth can largely be avoided so that you can continue to enjoy whatever activities bring you pleasure.

Fatigue

Fatigue is probably the most common cause of sports injuries. Our muscles need oxygen when they are working: the oxygen burns the food we eat to provide energy for the muscle to contract. The blood can carry only a certain amount of oxygen to a muscle at a given time, and overuse of the muscle through continued contraction depletes its available supply of oxygen. The muscle still needs energy, though, so the food, in the form of glucose, is burned without oxygen. When this

*See Ben E. Benjamin, *Sports Without Pain* (New York, 1979), for injuries common to each sport.

happens, lactic acid, a by-product of this process, accumulates. As a result of this acid-building, the muscle is less able to contract and perform. When fatigue occurs, the muscle needs to rest until the lactic acid is carried away and the supply of oxygen is returned. When the muscles are not allowed to relax, fatigue can become a chronic problem, setting the stage for injury.

Muscles, ligaments, tendons, bones, et cetera—all share the weight of the body. When fatigue sets in and the muscles give up their share of the workload, undue stress is placed on the other parts. When ligaments, for instance, are asked to do the work of muscles, they often strain and tear.

Excess Muscle Tension

Tension is produced by the contraction of the muscle fiber. We require a certain amount of muscle tension for life—tension allows us to move, to breathe, and it makes our hearts beat. But when a muscle is not being used it should relax. However, chronic muscle tension can accumulate over the years from poor physical habits, traumas from injuries, poor body alignment, emotional stress, and a variety of other causes. This excess tension creates muscular rigidity, makes movement stiff and unyielding, and diminishes blood circulation. The muscles become brittle and cannot absorb normal amounts of stress. As a result, they strain and tear more easily.

Lack of Flexibility

For certain activities we need the ability to twist, stretch, and bend into all kinds of positions. Without the maximum stretch and flexibility in your muscles, this is impossible, so injury becomes more likely. For instance, if you run and lunge to catch a ball, your hamstrings must stretch to complete this motion. If the muscle cannot stretch as far as it is being asked to, it will tear.

When you stretch a muscle, you are actually training the muscle fibers into a new elongated position. If you elongate your muscles slowly and regularly they will remain elongated for longer and longer periods of time. Few people have the patience to do this and instead force their muscles to get a quick result. When you force muscles to stretch they spring back to a tight position and often damage muscle or tendon tissue.

Improper Warm-Up

The right warm-up before any physically exerting activity is a must. Without it, nerve impulses are sluggish, reaction time is far below what it could be, heart and breathing apparatus fatigue easily, and cold, stiff muscles have no resilience. These conditions make us ripe for injury.

Strength

Strength (or lack of it) is the cause of injury only when you undertake an activity that your body is not strong enough to handle. Taking up a new activity without first building up the extra strength required can cause severe injuries, e.g., ruptured or torn tendons and ligaments. Your body often cannot absorb the added stress. If coupled with excess muscle tension, overbuilding your muscles can be as dangerous as not being strong enough. Extremely strong muscles are often rigid and inflexible and therefore can become injured frequently.

Your tendons stop growing when you reach adulthood. If you increase the strength of a muscle tenfold, so that you can lift great amounts of weight, you will be putting ten times more pressure on a tendon that can only minimally and slowly change its size to accommodate such increased stress. The result? Tendon strains.

Alignment

Good alignment of the bones, especially in the feet, knees, pelvis, and neck, can greatly reduce the occurrence of injury. If your body is properly aligned, your bones are in balance as they sit on one another, causing the least stress to the body. Examples of poor alignment are a neck that is constantly pushed forward or feet that turn out while the knees turn in. Poor alignment causes injury by placing stress on parts of your body that weren't built to accommodate it. If the bones of your feet are out of line, it is almost impossible to avoid injury to the ankle, knee, and hip, and if the pelvis and spine are out of line, back and neck injuries are more likely.

Alignment is not static. It is possible to have good alignment when moving. If your alignment is poor when you are moving, you are more vulnerable to injury. You can be born with problems that result in poor alignment, like scoliosis (a sideways curve of the spine), knock-knees, or flat feet. You can also develop poor alignment from poor habits or training, such as constantly pulling your shoulders back in a military stance, or tucking your pelvis to flatten your back, as many dancers do. These poor alignment habits make us tense in the neck, shoulders, and chest and make us prone to lower-back injuries. When your alignment is poor movement is inefficient. If you run in poor alignment your muscles will fatigue sooner because they are being asked to do more work than they normally should have to do. When the alignment is out of balance, especially during athletic activity, extra weight and stress are placed on the ligaments because the muscles are not being used efficiently. Let's look at a person who runs with his feet turned out. Every time his foot hits the ground, the foot is pointing to the side, and the knee is going forward. Because of this misalignment the weight is not going directly through the leg as it should, and the ligaments on the inner knee become overtaxed. In this situation, both the foot and knee become vulnerable to injury.

In most cases where an injury appears one day for no apparent reason, or in cases where a small ache gradually but continually worsens, poor alignment is a contributing cause. If your injury occurred during a normal or easy activity, such as picking up a ten-pound package or running half a mile when you regularly run three, your alignment may be out of balance.

Poor alignment leaves you more vulnerable to any injury. If you like being athletic, it's a good idea to try to change poor alignment. Misalignment of the neck, back, and to a lesser extent the legs, can be changed through training. Some of these retraining techniques are outlined in my book *Sports Without Pain*, but the best approach is to work with a realignment professional, such as an Alexander Technique teacher. Realignment of the knee and foot can be best accomplished with the use of orthotic devices discussed on page 38.

Muscle Imbalance

Muscle imbalance is destructive because it sets up an uneven tension and can throw your joint alignment off. Muscles work in pairs. When one set of muscles contracts, the opposite set releases its tension gradually and stretches. The body was meant to be used evenly so that one muscle balances another. For example, the spine can be pulled out of alignment by an uneven use and development of the muscles of the back. At the knee, an imbalance of the strength relationship between the muscles in the back thigh (hamstrings) and those in the front thigh (quadriceps) also invites injury.

If we don't develop the right and left sides of the body equally, the muscular balance of normal movement is disturbed. If one set develops disproportionately to the other, the paired muscles do not work efficiently, lose fluidity, and become distorted. Athletes tend to use their "good" side, and this tendency perpetuates itself, so the good side becomes stronger and the ignored side weaker. When exercising or playing at sports, it is best to use both sides, even if it looks and feels awkward at first.

Muscle imbalance presents its greatest danger after injury has occurred. If, for instance, one leg is injured, the tendency is to compensate by unconsciously using the other leg more. Two things now occur: the good leg is doing more work than it should, and the injured leg starts to atrophy (lose strength) especially in the tendon or muscle that was injured. Atrophy is one of the primary causes of reinjury, and we will discuss it more fully in the chapter on *Rehabilitation.*

Therapeutic exercise to re-establish the muscular balance after an injury is crucial, but it is often overlooked. Injuries arising from a failure to rebalance muscle strength are common and often more serious than the initial injuries.

4

Evaluating Your Injury

General Principles for Injury Evaluation

In the not-too-distant past, injury evaluation was more like guess-work than science. It has just been in the past fifty years that we have developed the tools to allow us to begin evaluating injuries with some measure of confidence. However, at the present time there are still many injuries that defy diagnosis. This book discusses common injuries that can be diagnosed and teaches you diagnostic tests that will help you determine what you have injured and how it can be treated.

For most of the injuries included in this book, one to three tests will be described to help you evaluate your problem. Before you jump into testing, you must first read the short introductory section on the body part you have injured, i.e., knee, shoulder, et cetera. After you have completed the reading, check the diagrams included with the section to locate the exact place of your injury. These diagrams will guide you to the appropriate section or sections that describe and test your injury. By carefully following the testing procedures for the structure you have injured, you will often be able to find the exact place that you have injured, or at least narrow the possibilities down to two or three places. Your findings may sometimes be confusing, especially if many different tests cause discomfort. This might mean that you have two or more injuries in the same shoulder or knee. It may also mean that the injury is quite complex, and you will need the care and/or advice of a physician. In many cases you will be able to figure out exactly what is wrong with confidence; but if you have any doubt about your findings, or if an injury is causing you serious pain, always see a doctor. Some areas of your body, such as your back, are too difficult or impractical to test by yourself.

When performing the various tests you will be trying to produce a feeling of pain *in the injured area.* If you are always in pain, the test will produce an increase in pain.

It is often helpful to irritate your injury slightly before you test it. If it hurts after you run, don't wait a few hours to test it—do it right after you run. It will be difficult to figure anything out if you felt pain two weeks ago, but waited until now, when you feel fine, to test it.

Do not continue to test your pain after you've discovered which test makes you hurt. Instead, it would be wise to avoid this movement as much as possible in your daily activities. People have a tendency to perform a movement that causes them pain continually, because they want to see if it still hurts. When you do this for a long period of time, say a few weeks, you only prevent yourself from healing. Test maybe once a day, but no more often than that.

The Tests and What They Tell You

There are three types of physical tests used in this book to help you determine what is injured. Understanding the meanings of these types of tests is essential. The first are *active movements,* in which you move a part of your body in a natural way. This is a preliminary test that often helps localize the general area of your pain. Active movements give you general information about your injury and define the kinds of physical movements that give you pain, such as lifting, walking, serving in tennis, hammering, running, and so on.

Movements against resistance (resisted movements) are isometric movements in which you use your muscles without movement through space. Putting your forearm on a desk and pushing down is a movement (pushing down) against resistance (the desk). This type of test is valuable because it allows you to test each muscle separately. *A movement against resistance is the best way to determine whether a muscle/tendon unit injury is present.* The muscle/tendon unit includes the muscle belly, the attachment of the muscle to the tendon, the tendon itself, and the attachment of the tendon to the bone. For example: You have a pain in the back of your thigh. You lie on your back on the floor with your lower leg on a chair and press your heel straight down into the chair toward the floor. If the movement caused you pain you would know that you had injured some part of your hamstring muscle—its tendon or its attachment.

In passive movements you go limp and someone else moves the injured part while you keep relaxed. The muscles around your injury do not do any work at all. *Passive tests are primarily used to determine injuries to the joints, ligaments, and bursas.*

If a ligament is injured, passive movements usually hurt while movements against resistance do not.

Active-movement tests are often misleading because the muscles, tendons, joints, bursas, and ligaments are all simultaneously involved in the movement. It is difficult to assess which is causing the pain. Passive and resisted movements differentiate the muscle/tendon unit from ligaments, joints, and bursas, and therefore allow you to determine the location of the injury more easily.

Evaluation by Touch

Feeling your muscles and tendons to locate your injury is often deceiving. If you squeeze any tendon, even if it is not injured, it can be painful. Another limitation of trying to evaluate by touching is that when you press on a muscle or tendon you may be pressing on other things as well—a bursa or a nerve—which will only confuse the picture. This is why just probing with the hands is usually not recommended as a tool for evaluation.

The X-ray Mystique

When X rays were first discovered at the turn of the century, it was as if magic had become a reality. Imagine seeing through people and photographing their bones! It revolutionized many aspects of medicine. At the same time, an all-powerful mystique about X rays was created and still persists today. The problem lies in the fact that most people think that X rays tell you a lot more than they actually do. X rays tell you *absolutely nothing* about the common injuries and pains that most people suffer from. To get a realistic view, let's look at what an X ray does not tell you about an injury and what it does.

An X ray does not tell you

1. if a muscle is injured.
2. if a tendon is strained or swollen.
3. if a ligament is sprained.

4. if a bursa is swollen.
5. if a joint is sprained or stiff.
6. if a joint has pain-producing adhesions.
7. if a nerve is inflamed.
8. if there is scar tissue.
9. if ligaments are loose.

Since most injuries occur to the ligaments, tendons, muscles, and bursas, X rays do not help the diagnosis very much. Because malpractice suits have become so common, physicians often feel they must take every possible precaution even when they feel an X ray is probably not necessary. Though X rays often fail to yield much-needed information and should not be depended upon or routinely given for all injuries, they are definitely necessary and valuable in some cases.

An X ray tells you:

1. if you have a severely broken or slightly fractured bone.
2. if you have a ligament or tendon completely torn away from a bone—*only* if it has taken a small piece of bone with it.
3. if a joint is loose, opening where it shouldn't, owing to the severe tearing of ligaments.
4. if there is a bony, loose body floating in a joint (a piece of chipped bone or calcified cartilage that has broken off and floats inside the joint).
5. if certain diseases are present (e.g., bone cancer, tuberculosis, osteomyelitis, and ankylosed spondylitis—a type of progressive spinal arthritis).
6. if the knee cartilage is torn (see Diagnostic Verification, p.109).
7. if a disc in the spine is displaced. (This test, a myelogram, in which dye is injected into the spinal canal, is less than 50 percent accurate.)

5

Treatment Choices

Many people don't know what to do when they have an injury. "Where do I go? What kind of treatment do I need—time, exercises, medicine, an injection, or what?" Not knowing what your choices are can leave you in pain for a long time. I worked with a woman once who loved cycling; for ten years long-distance biking had been a central theme of her life. It was her main form of exercise, her release from tension, and the centerpiece of her social life. For ten months she had been off the bike and miserable with a stubborn knee injury. She was doing exercises and not getting better. After I explained deep-friction therapy to her, she had nine treatments and was off biking again.

Though many people have given up hope, there is an answer to most pain problems. The trouble is that they often don't get an accurate diagnosis. What people also find so discouraging is that they have tried many treatments and have seen no improvement. If you have failed to connect with the right treatment, you may grow skeptical and reluctant to try something new. This chapter will explain a wide range of treatments and how they work. Some of these ideas are new in the United States and may seem rather strange. If you can, try to keep your skepticism in abeyance.

Certain symptoms automatically ought to ring bells of alarm. Sudden paralysis, rapid swelling, excruciating pain, loss of bladder or bowel control, severe numbness or weakness, and broken bones are all symptoms of potentially serious injuries. In all of these cases your only rational choice is to consult your physician immediately. But most injuries are not this dramatic; they develop over time and are annoying or painful but not incapacitating. Some disappear quickly of their own accord, while others are the seeds of lifelong pain problems. What follows are treatments that I know are effective.

Rest

Rest is probably the most common treatment of all. It's cheap and easy; unfortunately, it often doesn't work. Rest helps by taking the stress off the injured area. If you've injured your shoulder and you play tennis every day and irritate it regularly, it may never get a chance to heal.

Rest is usually effective when you've slightly strained a tendon or a ligament so that the fibers swell or tear only a small amount. Along with rest, it's important to move the injured body part but not to stress it. This is to prevent abnormal scarring and adhesions (described earlier on page 13), to promote blood circulation, and to help maintain normal strength to avoid atrophy. Atrophy, the breakdown in muscle tissue that occurs through disuse, occurs very swiftly. You can lose 20 percent of your tendon strength and muscle power within two weeks. Your tendons and ligaments can lose part of their mineral content with disuse. This further weakens their structure and makes them more vulnerable to reinjury.

Moving the injured part of your body should not be done to the point of pain. If you sprained your ankle, don't walk on it if it hurts but do flex and point the foot frequently throughout the day. Walk on it as soon as you can do so without pain.

Rest is frequently a very slow method of treatment. It is often frustrating, and so people tend to return to athletic activity too soon and reinjure themselves. Rest works for many injuries if you have the necessary time and patience, but in many cases, such as tendon ruptures, slipped discs, and poor scar-tissue formation in ligament injuries, rest is ineffective regardless of the amount of time given to it.

Heat

Heat has been used as a form of treatment for pain and injury for hundreds of years. What heat does is increase blood circulation in muscles, tendons, and ligaments that are close to the skin's surface. This speeds the healing process by increasing the supply of food and oxygen needed to repair damaged tissue. Heat is given in a variety of ways: with electric devices, water, and preheated materials such as hot packs. There are even special heat lamps that can heat muscles lying under the skin. Heat is useful for very minor strains where there is no swelling; for sore, tense muscles; and, in some cases, for temporarily easing pain. Application of heat *cannot* help painful scar tissue, inflammation and swelling, or pressure on a nerve from a ruptured disc. This is not to say that warm baths, hot packs, and heat lamps are not helpful adjuncts to effective treatment, but they are usually only marginally effective by themselves.

Ice Treatment*

Ice can be very effective as treatment, especially when applied immediately after an injury. Ice permits your body to heal quickly in two ways: it promotes even greater blood circulation than heat, and it numbs the pain so that you can move the injured area. The latter is beneficial because the best healing takes place when you actively move your injured part. Movement allows the new-forming tissue to remain pliable and healthy. The most amazing fact about this kind of treatment is that it drastically cuts the length of recovery time. Athletic trainers who use ice report that athletes who might have been out for the season can return to the field within one or two weeks after injury.

I can remember a young dancer who was anxiously rehearsing for his comeback performance with a large New York dance company. The day before the opening he sprained his ankle and it blew up like a balloon. He could barely walk and dancing seemed a total impossibility. I recommended that he put an ice pack on it for as many hours as he could stand it and intermittently move his ankle. Since this performance meant so much to him he kept the ice on almost continuously for twelve hours. To his surprise the next morning he could walk and that evening he was able to dance with very little pain. Although I wouldn't recommend this course of action to most people, ice can do some amazing things.

In order to benefit from ice you must use it correctly. For any of the techniques below the basic idea is the same: chill the injured area for about six to twenty minutes, or until it gets numb. Then begin to move it, starting with small movements and gradually increasing your range of motion. Remember to move *gently*, and without putting weight on the injury. When the numbness wears off and you start feeling the pain again, apply the ice and repeat the whole procedure. It is the movement part of the ice therapy that makes it so effective. Moving stimulates proper healing by increasing blood circulation and preventing abnormal scar tissue from forming.

*See "Cryotherapy—Putting Injury on Ice," by Ian Barnes, *The Physician and Sports Medicine*, vol. 7, no. 6, June 1979, pp. 130–36.

ICE TECHNIQUES

1. ICE MASSAGE: Massage the injured area directly with ice. You can use ice cubes or make an ice form that is easy to hold in a Styrofoam cup or a juice can. Work the ice gently on and around the injured part. Keep the ice moving for about twenty minutes before each set of exercises. If you leave bare ice on your skin in one place for too long, it can burn your skin.

2. ICE BATH: This technique is for the knees, ankles, elbows, or hands. Soak the injured part in crushed ice mixed with water for five to six minutes or as long as you can easily. If you have access to a whirlpool you can add ice to the water and soak the injured part in it. The ice water should be about 40°F.

3. ICE TOWEL: This is a good way to get to a large area, such as the back or the thigh. Soak a towel in 40°F ice water and place it on the injured area, resoaking as it begins to warm up. The ice towel is quite convenient because it can be used during exercise.

4. ICE PACK: This method is useful for injuries involving severe pain or swelling. Make a pack by putting crushed ice between two towels or filling an ice pack you buy at a drugstore with ice cubes. Leave it on for fifteen to twenty minutes. You can exercise the area either with or without the ice pack on. I find a regular ice pack the easiest method for most injuries.

WORDS OF CAUTION

Ice therapy is generally a safe and effective form of treatment, but as with any treatment, it is not recommended under certain conditions. If you have rheumatoid arthritis, Raynaud's disease* (a condition in which the fingers or toes become numb on exposure to cold), allergy to cold, diabetes, or a rheumatic disease, ice therapy is not recommended because the body reacts differently to lowered temperatures when these conditions are present. If you are in doubt, it's a good idea to check with your doctor first.

If you decide to use ice therapy, do not attempt any strenuous activity while you are numb from the ice. You could hurt yourself even more. The pain may be numbed but the injury is still there. In fact, a cold ligament or tendon is less flexible than it would be under normal circumstances and can be seriously injured, so be sure to move your injured part gently.

---

*Ice should not be used in Raynaud's disease because cold causes spasm of the small arteries in the sensitive areas. Fingers, toes, the tip of the nose, and the edges of the ears can develop gangrene owing to loss of blood supply from vascular spasm in this disease.

Deep Massage

Deep massage has been practiced for hundreds of years. Done by skillful practitioners with a functional knowledge of anatomy, it can be a great aid in the healing process. I am not referring here to light, pleasant massage. Massage, to be effective with injuries, must be somewhat deep in pressure and at times will be slightly uncomfortable, or even painful. Deep massage can help you heal faster by increasing blood circulation in the affected area. It can also reduce general tension in the body which, if unrelieved, can retard healing. It is indicated when there are minor muscle, tendon, or ligament strains and sprains as well as fatigue, soreness, and swelling.

Deep massage is not directly helpful in cases of disc problems, bruised nerves, severe sprains of ligaments deep inside the body, arthritis, fractures, and bursitis. It is an excellent postoperative therapy and can be a useful adjunct to any of the above conditions after they have been dealt with medically. When you are experiencing pain, your body makes many odd adjustments to compensate in an attempt to ease its discomfort. These adjustments often lead to increased muscle-tension levels and poor movement habits. The negative physical side effects often continue long after an injury is healed, and deep massage can help counter them.

Deep Frictioning*

Deep frictioning is a very precise form of medical massage developed by Dr. James Cyriax. It is remarkably effective in treating most muscle, tendon, and ligament injuries. It is ineffective, however, when the ligament or tendon lies deep within the body and cannot be easily reached with the finger.

It is done with no oils or creams and has no relationship to a pleasant, relaxing massage or to the deep massage described above. One or several fingers are placed on the skin at the exact point of injury. Pressure is applied while a constant back-and-forth action across the painful structure is maintained for anywhere from five to twenty minutes. This is somewhat painful at first, but the pain diminishes steadily as the treatment progresses.

Deep frictioning works by breaking down scar tissue that prevents proper healing within muscles, ligaments, and tendons. It also separates ligament-to-bone adhesions and allows normal healing to occur. Deep frictioning also increases the

*See James Cyriax and Gillean Russell, *Textbook of Orthopaedic Medicine*, vol. II (Baltimore, 1978).

blood circulation to areas that normally have very little blood supply; it accomplishes this through a mild, controlled trauma to tendons and ligaments.

I will never forget the first time I used deep frictioning. It was on a severe shoulder injury that was the result of a serious fall down some stairs. The woman I was treating had been in intense pain for seven months. She had tried medication, heat, and exercise—all to no avail. I had seen similar injuries but had not been able to treat them successfully because at the time I had not known about deep frictioning. After one session of frictioning my patient reported that her pain was half of what it had been. In three sessions she was almost completely better.

This case responded with such unusual quickness that I was astounded. I had not realized that deep frictioning would be such a powerful treatment tool. Most cases require nine to twelve treatments, which is still a remarkably short recovery time.

Deep frictioning requires a thorough and precise knowledge of anatomy. The practitioner must be able to pinpoint with his fingers the exact location of every muscle, tendon, and ligament attachment in the body. There are a limited but growing number of physical and other therapists in the United States who are trained in this technique. When deep frictioning is mentioned in this text it refers only to therapists trained in Dr. Cyriax's technique.

Injections

Many people want the quickest and easiest treatment method that's available, and often a well-placed injection of the proper medication works effectively and rapidly to accomplish this. However, other people prefer to avoid using injections until they have tried nondrug treatments.

In many injuries an injection is the only cure for pain. A structure that lies very deep in the body can be reached only by injection. Some injuries are simply not amenable to other types of treatment. For instance, an inflamed bursa is irritated by deep massage and is not helped by manipulation, but it can be successfully treated within a few days by injection.

INJECTING TO TEST A DIAGNOSIS
In cases where injections are desired, a test injection of a local anaesthetic will verify the diagnosis and help determine the exact location where the medication shot should be given. This substance (novocaine, Xylocaine, lidocaine) numbs the area to sensation, which should eliminate almost all of the pain within a few minutes.

Movements that previously resulted in pain are repeated several minutes after the injection. Assuming that the injection has been properly placed, an absence of pain means a correct diagnosis was made. On the other hand, if the painful sensations remain, the diagnosis was wrong or some additional areas require injection.

Although the pain returns within an hour or so, there can now be more confidence in the diagnosis. This diagnostic procedure is recommended when the site of the injury is unclear. Numbing injections are valuable when testing tendons, ligaments, muscles, bursas, and joints, except those in the spine above the lower back. Epidurals, described below, test disc injuries in the lower spine.

CORTICOSTEROIDS

There are many kinds of corticosteriods (hormone derivatives used in treating pain), but the kind most people are thinking of when they talk about corticosteroids is hydrocortisone. There is a lot of confusion about cortisone. First, there are two ways to take it. Cortisone pills taken orally for such problems as poison ivy or poison oak, colitis, skin rashes, and so forth, permeate your total system, stay in your body the entire time you're taking the medication, and can have many known side effects, most seriously, ulcers, decreased resistance to infection, increased blood pressure, and bone demineralization. Such serious medical side effects, however, usually don't occur unless cortisone is taken daily for at least thirty to sixty days.

Injectable cortisone that is used for injuries does not have the same effects on the body because it is never used daily over an extended period of time. When cortisone is injected it does not permeate your entire system. It affects just the area where it is placed and most of it is flushed out through the excretory system within twenty-four hours. Cortisone quickly works to stop inflammation and in injection form has practically no side effects. It does weaken some fibers, but this weakening is thought to be negligible unless many injections are given, thereby damaging a large amount of fiber.

Part of cortisone's bad reputation comes from the fact that it is used too frequently and indiscriminately. Almost any medication used in excess can be damaging. I used to be what I would call an anticortisone person. The major part of my concern for its dangers was based on prejudice and lack of evidence. I don't mind being proved wrong, and in this case I was. When I saw steroids being used conservatively I had to admit they could do miraculous things, which nothing else I had seen could accomplish. They can make a long-term chronic injury to a ligament, bursa, or joint pain free within a matter of days. Cortisone normalizes inflamed tissue, but it does it well only if it is injected into exactly the right places.

Usually the injection used is a mixture of local anaesthetic and a corticosteroid. The local anaesthetic has a twofold purpose. First, if the pain goes away it verifies that you got the right spot, and second, it dilutes the steriod.

Corticosteroids can take away inflammation from a painful area and also prevent the re-forming of unwanted scar tissue.

PROLIFERANTS*

A proliferant (also called a sclerosant) is a substance that causes the production of new tissue by stimulating connective-tissue cell reproduction. It is particularly useful in the treatment of ligament and tendon injuries, since the proliferant irritates the tendon or ligament into producing new cells. This new cell production strengthens the structure of the injured area. There are many different formulas of this substance in use by physicians throughout the world. One solution contains dextrose (sugar) and Xylocaine. Another one frequently recommended also contains phenol and propylene glycol. Dextrose, often used by itself, is a stimulant to connective tissue production. Phenol is both a sterilizing agent and a nerve block (blocks sensation to the nerve). Propylene glycol prevents contamination.

Proliferants are often effective where other treatments have failed. Unlike many drugs, they have no side effects and have a smaller drug content than an aspirin. Usually, proliferants are slower acting than other drugs because they stimulate your body to heal itself. They are especially effective in dealing with chronic lower-back pain and also in strengthening weak joints by shortening and thickening the ligaments that hold joints together.

Proliferants are a revolutionary form of treatment currently not well known in the United States. Until they were discovered it was believed that tendons and ligaments could not regenerate new cells and get stronger. Since this is such a new treatment in the U.S. it may be difficult to find doctors who are familiar with how it is used.

EPIDURALS

In some cases where there is a disc protrusion, epidural injections have been found to be effective. These are slowly given injections of local anaesthetic into the lowest portion of the spinal canal. They are thought to push the disc material off the nerve through increasing intraspinal fluid pressure. Various physicians claim success with them in a high percentage of cases. Why they work is really not clear, but one or two injections are often curative even in severe cases.

CHYMOPAPAIN

In November 1982 the FDA approved this new type of treatment for disc injuries

*The use of proliferants was originally developed by Dr. George Hackett in the 1940s.

developed by Dr. Lyman Smith. An enzyme that originates from the papaya is injected directly into the disc. Within a matter of hours the central portion of the disc disintegrates and relieves pain. It claims 80 percent effectiveness in certain types of disc problems. For instance, if pieces of disc have broken off into separate fragments, this treatment is not appropriate. Bear in mind that only 2 percent of lower-back injuries are thought to be from discs. This is a promising new alternative to surgery for about half of that group.

Medication

Oral medication is probably the most widely used medical treatment. Drugs do not have a high rate of success, but in some cases are very effective. Their greatest service is to get you out of pain while you are healing.

There are three types of medication that are commonly prescribed: anti-inflammatories, analgesics, and muscle relaxants.

Anti-inflammatory drugs such as Motrin and Nalfon are widely used when inflammation is a significant part of the injury. They give general relief while healing progresses. When injury is of the mild variety, they may be helpful, but in serious cases they often offer only temporary relief.

Analgesics or painkillers such as Codeine, Darvon, and Zomax, or stronger ones such as Demerol and Percodan, numb pain while you are getting better. They have no curative effect and may give a false sense that an injury is gone by masking the pain. This may encourage you to do things your body is telling you not to. On the other side, there have been times I wanted to thank God for giving me a pill to get me out of excruciating pain.

Muscle relaxants such as Valium and Robaxin mechanically relax the muscles and can be temporarily helpful for pain, particularly when stress is an important factor.

Medication usually permits symptomatic improvement, but generally doesn't get at the cause of the problem, which is not to say it isn't helpful in many cases. Medication is best when used as an adjunct to some more definitive treatment.

All oral medication may have some side effects, particularly because it must be taken daily over a period of time. It affects the entire body; it's systemic, not local to the injury site the way injection is. Drugs that were ingested may affect your digestion, bowel function, alertness, blood pressure, and so forth, and are potentially habit-forming.

However, medication has an important place in the treatment of injury, and when used judiciously, it can have great value.

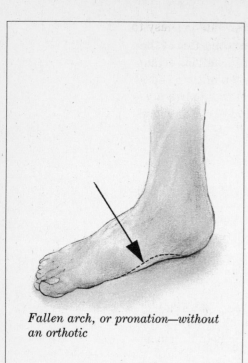

Fallen arch, or pronation—without an orthotic

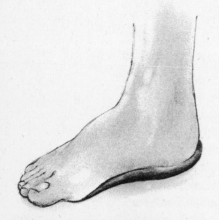

Aligned position—the arch supported by an orthotic

Orthotics

An orthotic is a custom-made molded arch support, made of leather, plastic, hard rubber, or even Styrofoam, that is inserted into your shoe; it helps to improve foot alignment so that your body weight is distributed properly throughout the foot. In this book we speak of pronation of the feet (fallen arches), which means that the arch rolls in toward the floor. Everybody's feet naturally pronate slightly to absorb shock during walking. When this pronation is excessive, it makes you vulnerable to injury to the ankle and knee.

If your foot is in an unaligned position when you walk, an orthotic can put you in the proper position. What it does is support the arch so that it cannot excessively roll in while walking or running.

Orthotics can help many other conditions. For example, they take pressure off the knee or lower-leg muscles. In other cases they will raise or support the heel, or realign or evenly support the small bones under the ball of the foot. Orthotics are used both as a treatment and as an effective method of prevention.

To obtain an orthotic you need to be fitted by a sports podiatrist. The best orthotics are made of leather or plastic, depending on your foot and the type of activity you do. When you have fully adjusted to them you wear them continually. To begin to adjust to your orthotics, wear them for an hour the first day while walking, and increase by an hour each day. Only when you can wear them comfortably all day are you ready to use them in sports activities. Several adjustments are usually required to obtain the perfect fit. If they do not fit you properly, they will not help and may even cause you some harm. Orthotics should not hurt when you wear them—if they do they are not properly fitted. Clearly explain to your doctor where they are uncomfortable, even if it takes ten visits. Your feet will feel better and the orthotics will be a pleasure to wear. It may take a little extra effort to find street shoes that fit your orthotics, but they are around. Special orthotics can be made to fit into high-heeled shoes, roller skates, ice skates, and ski boots. It is relatively easy to find running shoes and sneakers to fit your orthotics, but make sure the shoes are flat inside, without wedges or arch supports built into them. These built-in supports will negate or accentuate the effect of the orthotics.

Dr. Thomas Novella, a podiatrist, and Dr. Alan Weingrad recently developed orthotics that will fit into ballet slippers. Dancers often need these supports, which have until now been unavailable.

Manipulation

Manipulation of the joints, when performed by trained specialists, such as osteopaths, chiropractors, and physical therapists, can be enormously effective treatment. There are many theories as to why and how manipulation works, but no one understands it with any certainty. It is believed to restore the normal alignment of the bones, so that painful ligaments or nerves are not squeezed, stretched, or irritated, causing discomfort. It can be helpful in whiplash injuries, crippling, lower-back pain, adhesions of the shoulder, a loose body in the knee.

Before manipulation is carried out, it is essential to get a proper diagnosis. In certain instances this form of treatment can be so helpful that it seems miraculous, while at other times it can be of little value, or even dangerous.

The manipulation referred to in this book is medical manipulation. It is performed only after a thorough evaluation of the injury. Manipulation should not be performed where weakness, bladder disturbance, or pain during manipulation are present because it can increase your existing problems. Usually, manipulation is either rapidly effective or does not work at all.

Medical manipulation is often performed under some traction. If it is successful, the pain is eliminated or diminished immediately. Manipulation is considered an ineffective treatment if not successful after three to five visits.

DMSO (Dimethyl Sulfoxide)

DMSO is a solvent that is a by-product of wood. It has been used successfully by veterinarians in the treatment of horses and other animals for years. At the present time it has not been approved in the United States for use in humans by the FDA, although it is used extensively in Europe. DMSO comes in various strengths as a liquid, cream, or gel. Since it is a solvent it helps dissolve abnormal scar tissue and blood clots that are the result of a severe blow (hematoma); it seems to make many injuries heal more quickly. It has even been used intravenously for arteriosclerosis, a cardiovascular condition where the arteries are blocked.

DMSO penetrates the skin and moves into the body immediately on application. When applied to the skin along with other medicines it pulls the medicine in along with it. Although it is often used by itself, it is thought by some physicians to be very effective when combined with corticosteroid liquid applied to the skin. But until it has been approved by the FDA it is illegal to use as a pain remedy in this country.

Surgery

Although surgery should be the last resort in treatment choices, it should not be written off. The overwhelming majority of surgeons are highly skilled individuals dedicated to their work—we don't usually hear about them. What we do hear about are the few cases of greed or abuse. Surgeons quite naturally look at injuries with a surgical perspective because that's what they're trained to do.

Even though surgery is a consideration in only a small percentage of athletic injuries, it is the only solution at times. You should try all the alternative possibilities mentioned in this chapter if your doctor hasn't recommended immediate emergency surgery.

Although there are treatments included in this book that can often be more effective than surgery—such as particular neck and lower-back injuries, some kinds of arthritis, and severe ligament strains—there are emergencies that require surgery immediately. A slipped disc that presses on a nerve that controls your bladder and bowel functions, complete fractures of bone, or certain ligament and tendon ruptures need to be repaired quickly by surgical methods. And surgery is the treatment of choice for a severely torn knee cartilage, chronic dislocating kneecap, joint infections, and the like.

Never rush into surgery unless it's an emergency. Get two or three opinions from different physicians. If the risks of failure or of being worse after the operation are high, you may decide you would rather live with your pain.

When surgery fails it is usually for one of the following five reasons:

1. The diagnosis was incorrect or incomplete.
2. When the surgeon got inside there was too much damage to repair it all.
3. The physician was not experienced enough to do the operation properly.
4. The doctor did the best possible job but was limited by the present state of medical knowledge.
5. Painful scar tissue from a poorly healed surgical incision can cause continued pain after surgery. Skillfully administered postoperative corticosteroid injections into this tissue are helpful in abolishing pain of this type.

Though surgery can be effective in correcting an injury, any surgery is a trauma to the body. Deep massage and exercise can help you heal more quickly after surgery. They increase blood circulation and help restore normal muscle functioning. You should have professional guidance in implementing a massage or exercise program.

Traction

Traction means using weight to pull bones or joints apart. It is frequently used in neck and lower-back injuries that are associated with disc problems. The theory behind traction is that pulling the vertebrae apart creates an effect that sucks a protruding disc or a misaligned bone back into its proper place. There are times when traction is quite effective; however, we do not yet have an understanding of precisely how it works and why it works in some cases and not in others.

There are a number of theories on how to use traction best. Some theories suggest using small amounts of weight (five to twenty pounds) over long periods of time, while other theories suggest using a lot of weight (eighty to two hundred pounds) for brief periods of time. I prefer the latter procedure because the vertebrae are more effectively separated by greater amounts of weight.

Exercise

There are wide differences of opinion on the use of exercise as a treatment for injuries. Those in favor of it feel it is an effective tool in treating pain and injury, while those opposed feel that exercise alone is not effective as a treatment, though it has rehabilitative value when used in conjunction with other treatments. Practitioners using exercise as a treatment believe it works by increasing strength, flexibility, and blood circulation. Most proponents using exercise as treatment insist that exercises must be done daily in order to be effective at stopping pain. However, if the exercises are discontinued, the pain frequently returns. Opponents cite the above fact as proof that exercise does not cure injuries but only causes symptoms to abate temporarily. There is evidence to support both sides. What's important is to keep an open mind. Oftentimes exercise helps people when it's not supposed to. If it works, do it; if it doesn't, try something different.

II.

How to Find Your Injury

Part II of this book covers the most common injuries experienced by active people. The information in Part I gave you the background to understand the injuries, causes, and treatments dealt with here. If Part I is not fresh in your mind, you'll find it helpful to keep referring back to that earlier information.

The first thing you'll want to do is look up the body part that's injured—for instance, the knee. Read the brief anatomical introduction so you know what structures of the knee can be injured. The drawings that accompany each body part should guide you to your specific injury, which you can then look up. When you've looked up your injury you will find four sections discussing it.

1. "WHAT IS IT?"—this section describes what the injury is, where the pain is felt. It will describe and illustrate the specific anatomy of the affected ligament, tendon, bone, muscle, whatever.
2. "HOW AND WHY"—a typical progression of the injury and its possible causes are discussed.
3. "DIAGNOSTIC VERIFICATION"—this section shows you how to examine yourself and to test for the particular injury discussed.
4. "TREATMENT CHOICES"—here you will find both self-treatment suggestions and the various medical treatments for the specific condition.

For rehabilitation exercises, reconditioning, and prevention see Part III. The neck and back will be treated slightly differently from other body areas because evaluation of these injuries is much more complex.

45

6

The Foot and Ankle

Your feet and ankles take a lot of abuse. They are literally at the bottom of the pile—they have to support the weight of everything else in your body. In this chapter we will look at the most common ways that feet and ankles get injured. I have left out the more uncommon and horribly complex injuries because even the best physicians and therapists have a terrible time with them, and any discussion of them would be theoretical rather than practical, only adding our confusion to yours.

There are more bones in your feet than in your legs and back combined. Each foot has twenty-six joints. In the feet and ankles, fifteen different tendons can suffer tendinitis, more than ten different ligaments can become strained, and several bursas can become irritated. With so many parts it's easy to understand why the feet and ankles are so vulnerable to injury.

A host of other problems can affect the foot because of inherited structural problems in the formation of the bones. Different types of feet make people prone to different kinds of injuries. For instance, a high arch has half the

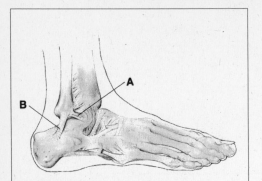

Foot and ankle, showing the anterior talofibular ligament (A), and the calcaneofibular ligament (B)

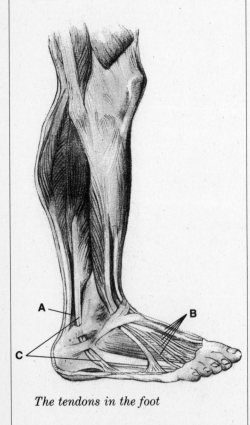

The tendons in the foot

weight-bearing surface of a normal foot; consequently, having a high arch creates problems in the heel and ball of your foot.

The foot and the ankle are dependent on each other for their safety. The ankle bones (or malleoli) are extensions of the bones of the lower leg. The inside of the ankle is the extension of the shinbone or tibia, while the outside ankle bone is the bottom of the fibula, the smaller bone in the lower leg which runs parallel to the tibia. These two bones are held together and are connected to the foot by strong ligaments.

The ankle joint is a hinge joint, moving primarily forward and backward. There is also some side-to-side movement that is vital to walking safely on uneven surfaces.

The ankles have ligaments on both the inside and outside which attach the ankle bones to the feet. The most troublesome ligament (A *above*) is the anterior talofibular. It tears partially or fully in 90 percent of all ankle sprains. This ligament goes from the front of your outer ankle bone to the talus bone, right next to it (see diagram). Another important ligament that is often torn is the one that goes from the outer ankle bone straight down to the outer heel (B *above*). Fortunately, the mass of ligaments at the inner ankle are very rarely sprained.

The most important tendon of the foot and ankle is the Achilles (A *below*), which attaches all the calf muscles to the back of your heel bone. There is also a group of tendons on the top of the foot (B *below*), which help flex the ankle and the toes, and an opposing group on the bottom of the foot, which facilitate pointing the toes and feet. Some of these tendons connect to muscles in the lower leg, while others connect to small muscles within the foot. In addition, there are tendons on either side of the foot (C and 2 on opposite page), which help you to move your foot from side to side. These tendons often become strained where they pass just behind the ankle bones.

In the next pages we cover the most commonly injured structures of the foot and ankle that account for about 85 percent of the injuries to this area.

LOCATING YOUR INJURY

Find the arrow in the drawing that corresponds approximately to where you feel your pain. This list will guide you to the name and page number of your injury.

1. Achilles Tendinitis   p. 196
2. Posterior Tibialis Tendinitis   60
3. Inner-Ankle Sprain   72
4. and/or 7. Anterior Tibialis Tendinitis   50
   or Extensor Hallucis Longus Tendinitis   56
5. Big Toe Joint Inflammation   54
6. Interosseus Strain   77
   (pain through the front of the foot)
7. See 4 above.

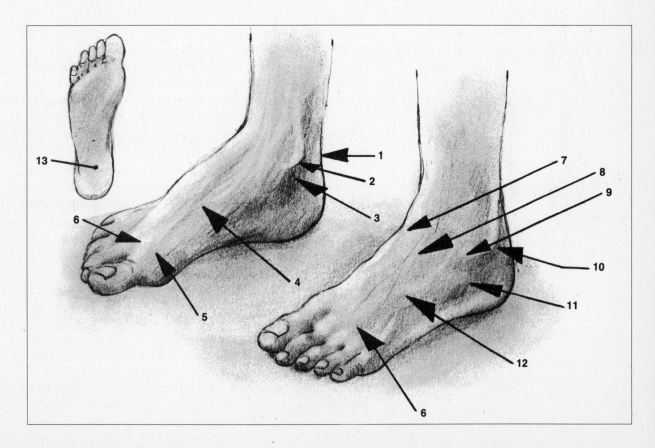

Important Note: Please read the full chapter on Rehabilitation before using the exercises described. In this way you can use them most effectively.

Pain on the Top of the Arch of the Foot
(Anterior Tibialis Tendinitis)

WHAT IS IT?

Anterior tibialis tendinitis is a strained tendon that can cause pain anywhere along the tendon from the inner arch of the foot (1) to about four inches above the ankle (2). In some cases only a small portion of the tendon is painful, but in others pain may be felt throughout its entire length.

If you flex your foot with your shoes and socks off, you can see the tendon sticking up in front of your ankle. If you trace it upward with your finger it will lead to its controlling muscle (A). If you trace it downward it crosses the center of the ankle and extends to the middle of the arch on the inside of the foot.

HOW AND WHY

The injury usually starts as a pain or ache on top of your foot just in front of the ankle. After a hard volleyball game, a long run, or a rigorous hike, an ache appears. Not too bothersome at first, but as the weeks progress it's there more often and for longer periods of time. You rest, it seems better—you're active, it gets bad again. When it becomes severe, just walking or flexing your foot hurts. Dancers frequently get this injury where the tendon

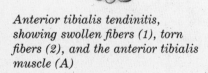

Anterior tibialis tendinitis, showing swollen fibers (1), torn fibers (2), and the anterior tibialis muscle (A)

meets the inside arch. Athletes, especially runners and basketball players, usually feel it in the tendon where it crosses in front of the ankle joint.

This tendinitis usually comes on over a period of time, but it can on occasion happen suddenly. In sudden cases a fall, jumping rope, or extra-strenuous activity, such as marathon running without adequate preparation, can cause this injury. In most cases the muscle controlling the tendon fatigues, too much stress is absorbed by the tendon, and injury occurs.

If your feet are pronated, which means your arches fall in, you will be more prone to this injury. Pronation greatly contributes to this strain because this tendon works to hold up the arch. It is therefore often stressed against unbeatable odds if the mechanical structure of the foot is out of balance. Severe tension in the lower-leg muscles is also a contributing factor to this injury because it subjects the muscles to early fatigue and the tendon to more stress than necessary. Ineffective warming-up procedures as well as running or jumping on concrete surfaces can make you prone to this injury.

DIAGNOSTIC VERIFICATION

Test 1
Flex your foot forcefully toward your knee against the resistance of your hand, as shown in the drawing. Your hand should be on the arch of your foot, not on your toes.

Test 2
Or, while standing, flex your feet, lifting the balls of your feet off the floor, and balance on your heels for a moment.

One or both of these tests should reproduce or increase your pain. To locate the exact area of your injury, press various places along the tendon while you hold your foot flexed.

If this doesn't seem to get it, try the sections on Extensor Digitorum Longus Tendinitis and Extensor Hallucis Longus Tendinitis (pp. 57 and 56).

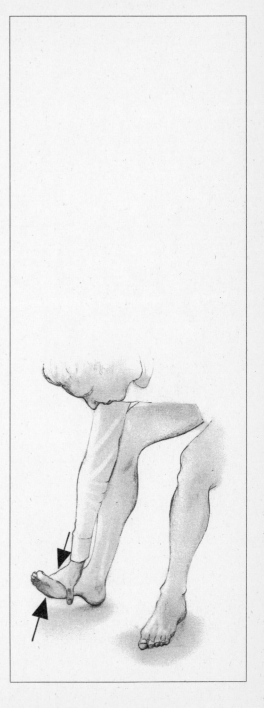

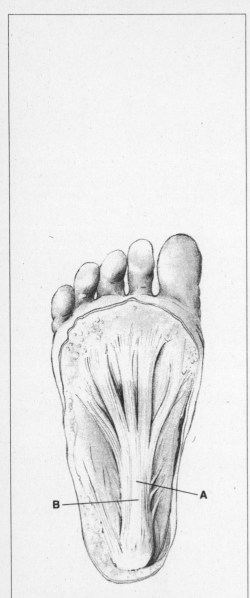

Plantar fasciitis. When the plantar fascia (A) is injured, you may feel pain at point B, and/or under the arch of the foot.

TREATMENT CHOICES

Self-Treatment

This particular tendinitis often takes a long time to heal because you use this tendon to walk, and thus you constantly irritate it. Rest and the ice treatment usually help over four to six weeks, but self-treatment of this injury is sometimes limited by the fact that it is often caused by a chronic mechanical imbalance of the foot. Don't take long walks, hikes, or runs if they cause pain. If severe pain lasts more than two weeks, seek medical treatment.

Medical Treatment

1. DEEP FRICTIONING: This treatment usually gives relief rather quickly because the tendon is easily accessible and near the skin, requiring only four or five treatments at most.
2. INJECTION: Corticosteroid injection is quick and usually effective. However, it is only recommended if other methods fail.
3. ORTHOTICS: An orthotic device, described on p. 38, can often correct the mechanical imbalance. See a sports podiatrist to see if an orthotic can help you. Removing the pressure with the orthotic is often curative as well as preventive.

Rehabilitation

See the Foot, Ankle, Shin, and Calf exercises on pages 266–67.

Pain Under the Arch of the Foot
(Plantar Fasciitis)

WHAT IS IT?

The plantar fascia (A) is a strong piece of tissue at the bottom of the foot. It functions like a big ligament, holding the bones of your feet in position. Starting at your heel, it runs under your foot and attaches across the ball of your foot. When a part of this fascia is strained, pain is felt at the front, inner part of the heel (B) and/or under the arch of the foot.

HOW AND WHY

This injury usually comes on gradually. Strain and discomfort are noticed at the front of the heel or the arch of the foot when you start an athletic activity. In severe cases, there is pain throughout the activity and/or afterward, or even while walking. In the more common, mild variety, the pattern that usually emerges is this: When you first get out of bed and walk in the morning there is brief pain under the foot for the first minute. The pain then ceases and only returns if you sit for a long period of time and then try to walk again.

When you rest at night, or even when you sit for a long period, the cells in the injured fascia begin to heal and repair themselves. However, this healing bond is very weak, so when you get up and walk and again place weight on the fascia, it tears repeatedly. That is why you feel pain when beginning to walk, and why the injury often lasts so long.

The most common cause of this injury is fatigue. It often happens to runners. The muscles of the feet get tired and cannot do their job in supporting the arch. The weight then falls onto the fascia, which is not built to handle it— thus the strain and tearing.

DIAGNOSTIC VERIFICATION

The location of the pain and the pattern of discomfort described above are the primary methods of diagnosis. Additionally, finger pressure with the thumb directly on the front, inner portion of the heel, as illustrated, creates a feeling of tenderness and usually causes pain.

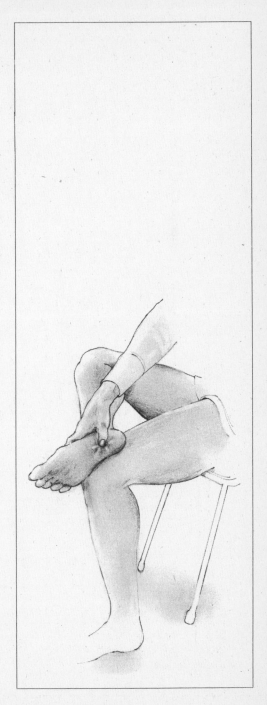

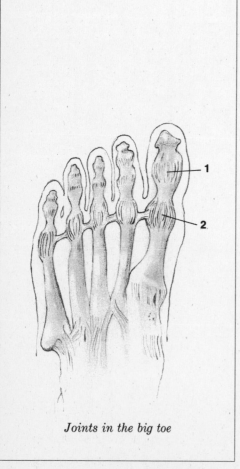

Joints in the big toe

TREATMENT CHOICES

Self-Treatment

The treatment of plantar fasciitis is quite simple. You must avoid any stress on the fascia until it is sufficiently healed. To do this, all you need do is wear a heel lift in all your shoes. It must be thick enough to take the weight off the injured fascia. Experiment with adhesive foam (which you can get at a drugstore) until you find the right height and feel no pain when you begin to walk. What is essential is that you *always* wear the lift. Forgetting for one day can nullify the whole treatment. This means that if you get up to go to the bathroom in the middle of the night, you must put your shoes on—and there must be no going barefoot at all. Continue the treatment for about three months—the fascia is a slowly healing structure. Avoid athletic activity for a week to ten days to allow the healing to begin. After this time activities are fine as long as you are wearing your lift.

Sometimes it is difficult to devise a successful lift yourself because of other factors in the construction of your feet (e.g., a severely fallen arch). In such cases it is best to see a sports podiatrist to be fitted for an orthotic, molded arch support. This should relieve your symptoms if you wear it faithfully. If orthotics are indicated in your case, they may also help prevent a recurrence in the future.

A word of caution: Don't stretch your calf, do high jumping, or sprint during the healing period.

Medical Treatment

INJECTION: Corticosteroid or proliferant injections are effective within two weeks.

Joint Pain of the Big Toe
(Traumatic Inflammation)

WHAT IS IT?

When the big-toe joint is injured, the inner lining of the joint is irritated and inflamed. Although the pain can be quite sharp when it is strongly forced in either direction, discomfort is commonly felt as a general aching sensation in the big-toe joint. The large toe has two joints (1 and 2 in the illustration), in contrast to the other toes, which have three. Usually it is joint 2 that gets injured because this joint supports more weight than any of the others.

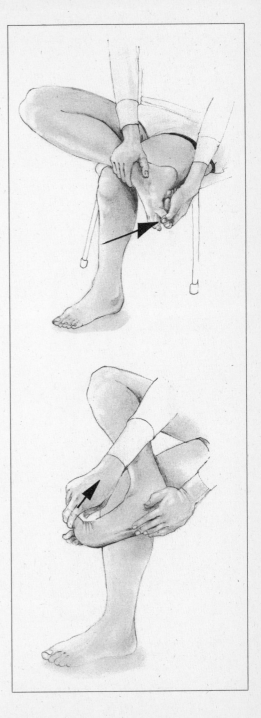

HOW AND WHY

The joint may hurt during walking, running, jumping, or all three. In some cases it may ache only after activity. It seems to come and go with no rhyme or reason, and it has a tendency to recur if the joint suffers additional abuse.

I have known many a dancer with this persistent injury, especially those who dance on toe. Let's face it, most of us were not born to stand on our toes, and when we do, most of the weight falls on the big one, which gets inflamed in some with regularity.

This condition can result as well from stubbing your toe or from athletic activity with poor alignment of the legs and feet. Tight, pointed shoes can also cause irritation of the big-toe joint. It is generally brought on by running or jumping on hard surfaces in combination with an extreme drop of the arches of the feet (pronation).

DIAGNOSTIC VERIFICATION

Bending your injured toe joint forcefully foward and downward and/or backward (as illustrated) is usually painful.

TREATMENT CHOICES

Self-Treatment

Rest will usually help, but it takes several months of no vigorous activity. Don't walk barefoot or wear high-heeled shoes. Instead wear round-toed shoes which don't push your big toe inward.

Medical Treatment

1. STRETCHING: In an old, chronic inflammation, adhesions of scar tissue may have formed inside the joint. In these cases, forceful stretching of the joint by a trained therapist is often helpful.
2. INJECTION: One or two injections of small amounts of cortisone usually cure the immediate problem. However, if the cause is not found and corrected, it may recur over and over again.
3. ORTHOTICS: An orthotic device to alleviate pressure on your toe joint is usually both a good treatment and preventative measure.

Pain on the Top of the Foot Between the Front of the Ankle and the Big Toe
(Extensor Hallucis Longus Tendinitis)

WHAT IS IT?

This tendon strain often occurs at the front center of the ankle but can be painful anywhere along the tendon indicated in the drawing. The extensor hallucis longus muscle allows you to flex and pull up your big toe. It lies underneath the muscle just to the outside of your shinbone, but its tendon (A in the drawing) is clearly visible on top of the foot. The tendon runs from the big toe diagonally across the foot, disappearing above the center ankle, where the muscle begins. Just lift your big toe up toward your knee and you will see the tendon stick out.

HOW AND WHY

This injury can happen suddenly or gradually as a fatigue phenomenon. It can also occur in a fall in athletic activities, where the toe is pointed down into the floor. The arch of your foot is stretched too far and the tendon tears. But

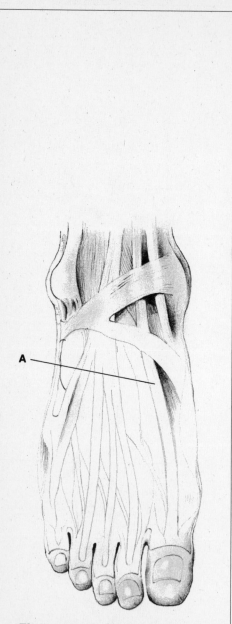

A

The extensor hallusis longus tendon (A)

it's more frequent in dancers who balance on the balls of their feet or their toes for extended periods.

DIAGNOSTIC VERIFICATION

Test
Place your injured foot on the floor and put your thumb on your big toe, at the base of the toe. Now try to lift that toe off the floor while resisting lifting by the pressure of your thumb (as illustrated). That should cause you pain. If not, try tests for Anterior Tibialis Tendinitis (p. 50) and Extensor Digitorum Longus Tendinitis (see below).

To locate the exact spot, feel along the tendon with the toe flexed up. It will be quite tender.

TREATMENT CHOICES

Self-Treatment
If it's minor, ice with a few days' rest will often take care of it. In between ice applications, point and flex the toes forty or fifty times in a row.

Medical Treatment
1. DEEP MASSAGE: This treatment, done somewhat forcefully over the entire foot, is effective.
2. DEEP FRICTIONING: This procedure works well with this injury, and usually only two or three treatments are necessary.
3. INJECTION: Corticosteroid injection is effective as well.

Pain on the Top of the Foot
(Extensor Digitorum Longus Tendinitis)

WHAT IS IT?

The extensor digitorum muscle begins just below the knee at the outside of your leg. It travels down the outside of

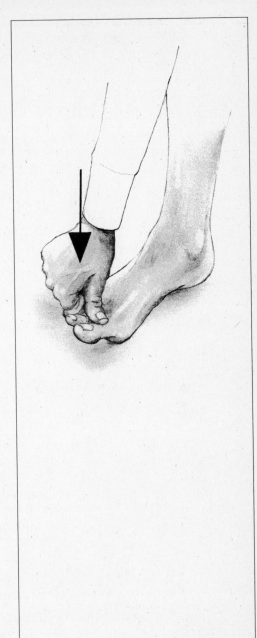

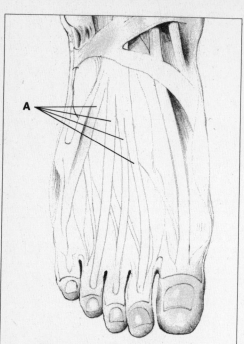

The extensor digitorum longus tendons (A)

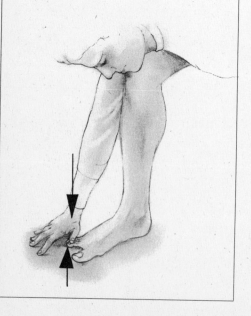

the leg, crosses over the front of the ankle, and then branches out to form four separate tendons (A), which attach to each of your four outer toes. This muscle-tendon unit enables you to lift up all four toes. When you injure one or more of these tendons you will feel pain anywhere along the tendon from the toes to slightly above the center ankle.

HOW AND WHY

You can injure these tendons when dancing, when you receive a direct blow during kicking sports, or when in utter frustration and fury you kick a piece of furniture. Sometimes this tendinitis comes on slowly as a result of compensating for another injury, such as Achilles tendinitis, or knee pain.

DIAGNOSTIC VERIFICATION

If this injury is severe, it hurts to pull the toes back, but the definitive test is to pull your toes back against resistance.

Test
While sitting, place your foot flat on the floor. Place your thumb on each of your small toes, one at a time, at the toenail, and press down firmly while at the same time trying to lift your toe against your thumb's pressure, as illustrated.

NOTE: *This injury is often confused with cruciate crural ligament sprain. Check p. 59 to try to differentiate the two.*

TREATMENT CHOICES

Self-Treatment
Try rest and ice for a week, and don't do any kicking or running. If you are not better, seek some therapy.

Medical Treatment
1. DEEP FRICTIONING: This is usually an effective treatment.
2. INJECTION: Corticosteroid injections are effective also.

Pain on the Top of the Foot Near the Ankle
(Cruciate Crural Ligament Sprain)

WHAT IS IT?

This sprain is felt as pain on the top of the foot. Pain can be felt anywhere along the ligament. The tendons that lift the toes are held in place by this braceletlike ligament (A) that runs across the top of your foot from the inner ankle to the outer ankle.

HOW AND WHY

This ligament can be injured by all kinds of common and strange falls, from falling down a flight of stairs to tripping in a hole. It can also come from a blow to the instep, which is common in contact sports, such as soccer and football. It is rarely caused directly by fatigue or alignment problems. Because of the ligament's relationship to the tendons controlling the toes, the tendons may become injured as well. The foot usually swells and is very painful where the tear is (see illustration).

DIAGNOSTIC VERIFICATION

Test
Perform test on page 58. Note how much pain, if any, results. Now, press your thumb firmly along the ligament, as illustrated. If this causes more pain than lifting your toes did, you probably have injured the ligament rather

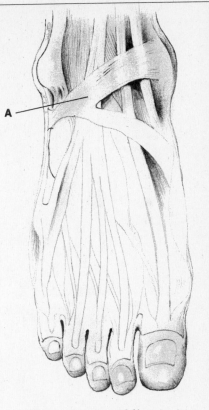

The cruciate crural ligament

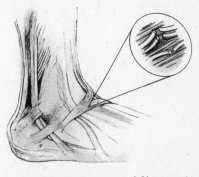

Injured cruciate crural ligament

than the tendons beneath it; to doublecheck, read the section on Extensor Digitorum Longus Tendinitis (p. 57).

TREATMENT CHOICES

Self-Treatment

Flex and point your toes ten to fifteen times at several intervals during the day to prevent poor scar-tissue formation.

Try not to do too much walking and use ice (pp. 31–32) as much as you can.

Medical Treatment

1. DEEP FRICTIONING: This treatment works well if the tearing is not too severe.
2. INJECTION: A widely peppered corticosteroid injection is curative within a few days.

Pain Just Behind the Inner Ankle
(Posterior Tibialis Tendinitis)

WHAT IS IT?

This tendon strain often occurs at the same time as shin splints (p. 198). This happens because the tendon (A) is the extension of the posterior tibialis muscle, which is injured when you have shin splints. Luckily, it isn't very difficult to distinguish between these two injuries. Shin splints are indicated where pain is felt higher up at the inner part of the leg (1). If you feel pain just above or behind the inside of the ankle—or on the foot itself several inches in front of the ankle—(2, 3, or 4), you have tendinitis. Although the pain tends to be most intense behind and above the inner-ankle bone, it can occur at any point along the tendon.

HOW AND WHY

This injury usually develops slowly. At first it feels like an irritation somewhere behind the inner-ankle bone. As the

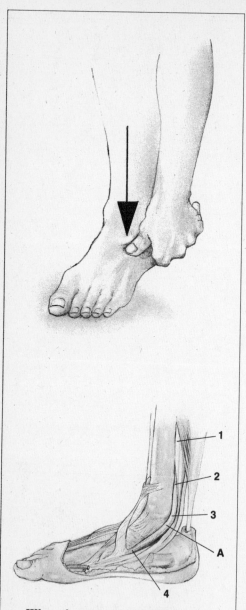

When the posterior tibialis tendon (A) is injured, pain is felt at points 1, 2, 3, or 4.

demands of exercise activity increase, it gets progressively worse until, in some cases, it's debilitating. In severe cases where trauma occurs suddenly, such as a fall, the inner ankle can become quite swollen and blow up like a balloon. The swelling often encompasses a large area, making it difficult to reach a correct diagnosis easily.

This injury is largely caused by fatigue in running and jumping sports. Lack of proper warm-up can contribute to it, as can fallen arches. If you have fallen arches, the tendon muscle unit must constantly strain to compensate for the fallen arch. Since the tendon was not designed for this constant extra stress, it is inevitably injured.

Severe traumatic injuries are common in soccer, resulting from two players simultaneously hitting the ball with the inner sides of their feet.

DIAGNOSTIC VERIFICATION

In this injury pain is usually felt while walking, when rising on the ball of the foot, or while pointing the foot. But most painful is the inward movement of the foot against resistance.

Test

Sit in a chair and cross your injured foot over the other leg just above your knee, as shown. Place the heel of your hand on your big toe joint and try to push the big toe up toward your head with all your strength. Push down with the heel of your hand with equal strength so that you stress the tendon without actually moving. If this hurts, you have posterior tibialis tendinitis.

TREATMENT CHOICES

Self-Treatment

First, it's important to stop doing activities that give you pain. Certain sports activities may be fine, while others may cause pain. If you run or dance, do it only for an amount of time that it is comfortable and does not cause

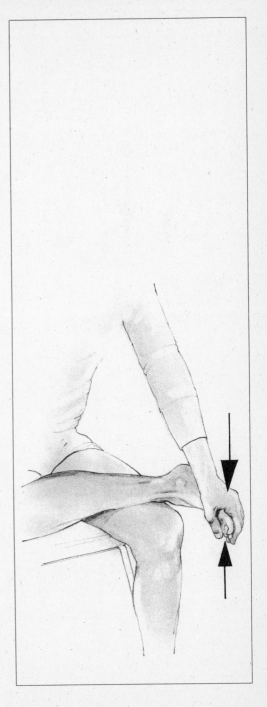

you pain. Remember that when tendons are warmed up, pain is often masked, so take it slowly at first.

Rest and ice treatment with the rehabilitation exercise below will help if the strain is not too severe. It's common for this injury to recur if it isn't treated properly and you don't take the proper measures to prevent it from recurring. This means not returning to full activity too soon, warming up thoroughly before vigorous sports, and correcting your foot alignment, through exercises or orthotics, if needed.

Medical Treatment

1. DEEP FRICTIONING AND DEEP MASSAGE: The most common site of this injury is where the muscle joins the tendon. A very effective treatment is deep frictioning used in conjunction with deep massage of the surrounding muscles to aid circulation.
2. ORTHOTICS: If you have fallen arches, get orthotic devices for your shoes. These devices protect the posterior tibialis muscle and tendon from further strain, which often makes orthotics the most crucial component of the treatment.
3. INJECTION: Corticosteroid injections should help if the above don't work for you.

Rehabilitation

See the Foot, Ankle, Shin, and Calf exercises, especially the Inner-Ankle Lift, p. 267.

Pain Just Behind the Outer Ankle
(Peroneal Tendinitis)

WHAT IS IT?

Peroneal tendinitis involves a strain and partial tearing of some of the fibers of one or both of the peroneal tendons (A and B). The pain can be felt at a number of places, such as the outside of the leg just above the ankle, under the

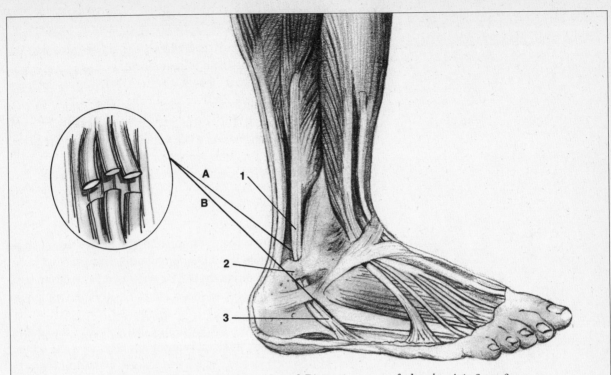

When the peroneal tendons (A and B) are torn, you feel pain at 1, 2, or 3.

outer ankle, or at the outside of the foot below the ankle (1, 2, or 3). However, the most common place for this injury is very close to the ankle bone.

The two peroneal muscles begin at the outside of the lower leg just below the knee and travel down toward the ankle. Their tendons begin just above the ankle. They wrap around the back of the outer ankle bone in a little groove. These two tendons are called the peroneus longus (A) and peroneus brevis (B). Their major function is to stabilize your leg when walking so that your ankles don't wobble and give way. The longus ("the long one") helps you to move your foot out to the side when the foot is pointed, while the brevis ("the short one") lets you move the foot out to the side when it's in a flexed position.

These tendons can be touched easily by feeling just behind and above the outer ankle bone if you flex the foot and turn it outward.

Part of the difficulty in evaluating this injury is that when these tendons tear they are often mistaken for a minor ankle sprain, because the pain is felt in a similar place. In fact, these tendons are often sprained along with the ankle, and are frequently missed during a diagnosis.

HOW AND WHY

Often this injury occurs from common accidents, such as stepping in a hole when running, sliding into second base, or being fouled in basketball or soccer, or any other accidents involving your ankle turning with your foot under you.

Ballet dancers get this injury frequently. Years ago, pointing the foot while moving it slightly outward (called *sickling* out) was considered more beautiful than a straight pointed foot. Dancers who still believe this point their feet in this way, placing constant strain on these tendons and making them very vulnerable to this injury.

If you have pronated feet (fallen arches), you are also vulnerable to this injury. When the arch is dropped, the outer muscles and tendons strain to maintain some semblance of balance. These factors speed fatigue and strain.

DIAGNOSTIC VERIFICATION

Although it often hurts just to walk or rise up on the ball of the foot when you have strained one of the tendons, moving the foot outward against a resistance usually creates the most pain.

Test 1

Sit in a chair and cross your legs with your injured ankle resting on your other knee. Point your foot and hold it there. Wrap your hand around the outside of your foot,

Test 1

holding on to the small toes, as shown. Now with your hand try to pull the front part of your foot forcefully up toward your head while offering resistance to this movement by pushing your foot down toward the floor. This tests tendon A (the longus).

Test 2

To test the other tendon (B), the brevis, take the same position, but this time keep your foot flexed (back toward your knee) the entire time, as shown. Push as hard as you can against the resistance of your hand—as illustrated.

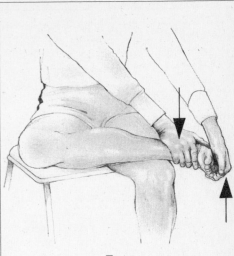

Test 2

TREATMENT CHOICES

Self-Treatment

As with many of the injuries we've discussed, strenuous activity should be stopped immediately and ice therapy applied, using the rehabilitation exercises below. If it's a very minor strain, a bit of rest sometimes does the trick. If the tendinitis lasts more than a few weeks, medical treatment is recommended.

Medical Treatment

1. DEEP FRICTIONING: This treatment works well for the longus tendon, which is near the surface.
2. INJECTION: If the tendinitis is in the brevis tendon, which lies underneath the longus, corticosteroid injection is the most effective treatment when the condition is chronic.
3. ORTHOTICS: If stress on the tendons is relieved while walking, you will be injured less frequently. Special orthotics for ballet dancers have recently been developed by Dr. Thomas Novella, a New York podiatrist, and Dr. Alan Weingrad.

Rehabilitation

See Foot, Ankle, Shin, and Calf exercises, especially the Outer-Ankle Lift, p. 267.

Outer-Ankle Sprain

WHAT IS IT?

I have rarely met an active person who has not sprained his or her ankle at least once. Along with lower-back problems it's probably the most common injury. A sprained ankle involves the partial or total tearing of ligaments at the ankle. About 95 percent of all sprains occur to the ligaments on the outer side of the ankle. The seriousness of this injury varies considerably. In a minor sprain only some of the fibers tear, but in major sprains at least one of the outer ligaments tears completely in half.

An outer-ankle sprain involves the strain of one or two

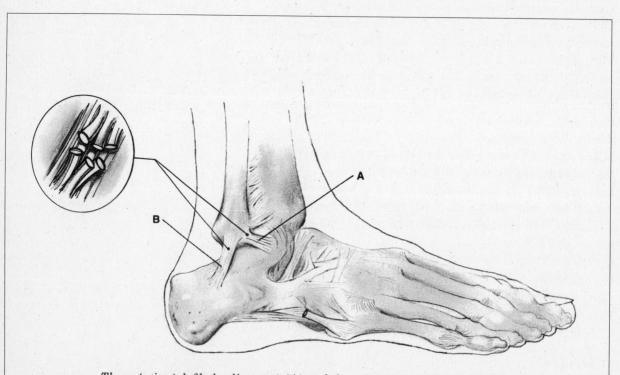

The anterior talofibular ligament (A) and the calcaneofibular ligament (B)

ligaments (A and B). In most cases ligament A is affected, and in severe sprains both ligaments A and B can be torn. Ligament A extends from the front of the outer ankle bone to the bone in front of it. Although it's only about one inch in length, it is an important stabilizer of the foot. It supports the outside of the foot and helps prevent your ankle from falling over.

Ligament B extends from the bottom of the outer-ankle bone straight down to the heel bone. It aids ligament A in stabilizing the outer ankle.

When one or both of these ligaments tears or becomes stretched, your ankle becomes unstable. Ligament B doesn't usually tear unless ligament A is torn also.

HOW AND WHY

You can sprain your outer ankle in two ways. Usually it happens during athletic activity and involves a severe, sudden trauma, such as coming down from a shot in basketball or a jump in dancing and landing incorrectly; crashing into somebody in soccer; sliding into second base; or tripping on some uneven ground while running. There is severe pain and sometimes a disconcerting "snap" is heard. It takes a few hours for the swelling to occur and the pain to worsen. When this happens it is very difficult to walk.

In other cases, the sprain is not immediately apparent. In the heat and excitement of activity, a slight falling over on the ankle is barely noticed; you recover your balance automatically, without missing a step. An hour or so later, a nagging pain with or without swelling begins to appear. It often remains just a slight irritation, which gets worse over the next few days as you use your ankle more.

In a mild sprain, the pain pattern is often irregular, causing pain at the beginning of activity and several hours after activity has stopped. This same pattern also emerges when a severe ankle sprain does not heal properly. The pain from an old, chronically sprained ankle is generally caused by scar tissue that is malformed during the healing process. The ligament grows on to and adheres to the bone it is supposed to glide over. Strenuous activity then tears this weak and unwanted scar tissue, causing a seemingly endless cycle of pain, no pain, pain, and no pain. It's a nasty problem that can continue for years if not properly treated.

What activities or conditions lead to sprained ankles? Poor alignment of the bones of the feet—arches that tend to drop and knees that turn in—make you prone to ankle sprains. High arches, which make you less steady, and excessive flexibility at the ankle, which comes from loose or stretched ligaments, increase the likelihood of your falling over your ankles and spraining them. If you have severely tense lower legs they are less able to adapt to changes in the ground surface, increasing your vulnerability to injury. Another cause of ankle sprains can come from an uneven muscular development in the lower leg.

Though many people like to wear them, platform or high-heeled shoes create an instability that can cause ankle sprain. And, of course, you could be doing everything just right, slip on a banana peel or ice, or have someone bang into you, and end up with a terrific sprained ankle.

DIAGNOSTIC VERIFICATION

Within a few hours after you sprain your ankle, the swelling and pain are often so severe that they can make an exact diagnosis difficult for you until the swelling begins to go down. If an ankle is badly sprained it can swell out to the size of a grapefruit. There are three grades of sprains: mild, moderately severe, and extremely severe. In reaching a diagnosis you can usually judge the extent of the sprain by the severity of the pain. However, there is an exception to this.

In the extreme sprains where the ligament totally ruptures, there is sometimes no pain at all after a short time. Although the pain usually subsides quickly, the ankle feels extremely unstable, since a major ligament is now useless.

When swelling and pain are present, get an X ray before fooling around with it. You could have a broken bone.

Test

Let's assume you've sprained your right ankle. Cross the right lower leg over the left knee and place your right hand on your right inner ankle bone. Place your left hand under the sole of your foot, wrapping your fingers around your small toes. Now, relax your foot and push down on your inner ankle with your right hand, and at the same time pull the front of your foot forcefully toward your head with the left hand, as shown. If you have sprained your ankle, that should be painful.

If your sprain is very mild, or is an old, chronic one, you

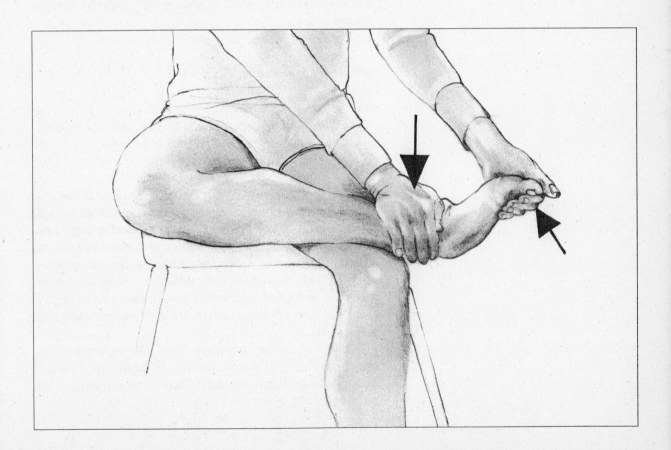

will need to give your foot a jerk up toward your head with your left hand after you have it in the stretched position. This should reproduce your pain.

A sprained tendon just behind the ankle (peroneal tendinitis) is sometimes mistaken for a mildly sprained ankle because this tendon passes very close to the ligament that is usually sprained. Additional confusion comes from the fact that the pain is similar in both injuries.

In cases of severe ankle sprain, one or both of the peroneal tendons are often stretched and torn along with ligaments of the ankle. What often happens is that the ligament heals but pain remains, and this pain is from an undiagnosed and untreated sprained tendon. If it's been a month and it still hurts behind or below your outer ankle, this may have happened to you. Check page 62 for this tendon injury.

TREATMENT CHOICES

Self-Treatment

When you sprain your ankle, stop your activity immediately, elevate your leg, and wrap it in ice. See your doctor to check if you have broken any bones or ruptured your ligament completely. If it isn't broken, rest, use the ice treatment, and elevate your leg as much as possible. As soon as you can move your ankle, flex it, point it, and circle it in both directions many times throughout the day, always keeping it elevated while suspended in the air. This will prevent adhesions of scar tissue from forming.

Don't begin to walk on it until there is only mild discomfort. Be careful not to rush into any sports or dance activities, for a resprained ankle is often worse than the original.

In mild and even in severe cases, the self-care treatment described above can promote successful healing. This generally takes two to six weeks, depending on the severity of the injury.

These instructions do not apply when the sprain is an

extremely severe one. If it is, you should be under the care of a physician.

Medical Treatment

1. DEEP MASSAGE AND DEEP FRICTIONING: When performed by a trained therapist, deep massage is effective in both mild and moderately severe cases. Massage, applied directly to the foot and leg, can reduce the swelling in the area and help to feed in fresh blood for healing. When massage is combined with deep frictioning of the damaged ligament, treatment is even more effective. The frictioning stimulates the healing of the ligament while preventing unwanted scar tissue from taking hold.

2. MANIPULATION WITH DEEP FRICTIONING: In old, chronic cases, the adhesive scar tissue must be separated from the bone and then must be prevented from re-forming. This can be easily accomplished by a skillful therapist who softens the scar tissue with a prolonged friction treatment, followed by a forceful manipulation of the ankle, which stretches the ligament and gently separates it from the bone. If done properly, this treatment needs doing only once or twice. It should be followed by several additional deep-friction treatments and daily exercising of the ankle to prevent scar tissue re-formation.

3. INJECTION: Corticosteroid injection is an effective treatment in both chronic and moderately severe sprains. The medicine must be injected into *all* of the tender parts of the ligament in order for it to be fully effective.

   When there is an overstretching of the ligament, injections of proliferant can tighten and strengthen the sprained ligament.

4. SURGERY: When the ligament fibers are totally ruptured, surgery is very often effective. However, the longer one waits after the accident, the less likely the success of the surgery, because the ligament tends to heal by adhering to anything near it. In surgery of

this type, the torn ends of the ligament are sewn together. Results from this type of surgery have been very successful.

5. CASTING AND STRAPPING: When an ankle sprain is extremely severe, involving total rupture of the ligament, casting or strapping techniques are usually used.

In casting, the foot is held in an aligned position and a plaster cast is applied to the foot and lower leg, remaining in place for two to three months. It is hoped that scar tissue will form between the ends of the ruptured ligament, restoring it somewhat to its natural function. With a little luck, this sometimes happens. But frequently there is poor scar-tissue formation, and discomfort and slight swelling persist for a very long time; the ankle never quite feels the same.

Other physicians use a strapping technique where the foot is securely taped in the aligned position. This allows for more freedom of movement in the foot and ankle than the casting technique. The goal here is the same: that the ends of the ligament will approach each other and grow together with scar tissue, but the ability to move usually allows for a better success rate.

If the strapping technique is employed, along with a proliferant injection and a gentle exercise program, the results are usually even better.

Rehabilitation
See the five Foot, Ankle, Shin, and Calf exercises, pages 266–67.

Inner-Ankle Sprain

WHAT IS IT?

An uncommon version of the sprained ankle involves ligaments on the inner side of the ankle. This fan-shaped liga-

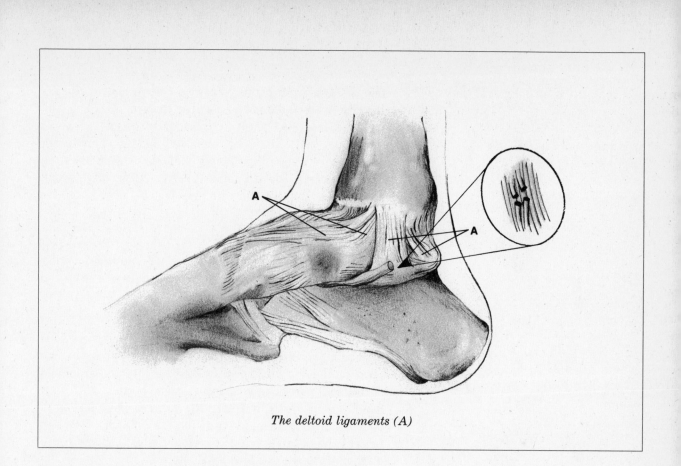

The deltoid ligaments (A)

ment complex (A) begins on the lower half of the inner ankle bone, and bands of the ligament fan out and attach to the heel and the bones in front of the ankle. In an inner-ankle sprain, one or more of the bands of this powerful set of ligaments tears. However, it is extremely rare for them to tear in half totally—that is, to rupture completely. The pain is felt directly below the inner-ankle bone, and either slightly in front of or slightly behind it, and radiates downward.

HOW AND WHY

It's easy to picture accidents that cause outer-ankle sprains, but inner-ankle sprains are harder to visualize. In this uncommon sprain, it's usually an awkward, bizarre fall, a freak accident, or a blow to the outside of the leg that causes your ankle to collapse inward. Swelling and pain increase over the next several hours, after one of these falls, and walking becomes very painful. This sprain occurs more frequently in older individuals than in young people because the ligaments tend to stiffen up slightly and become more brittle with age.

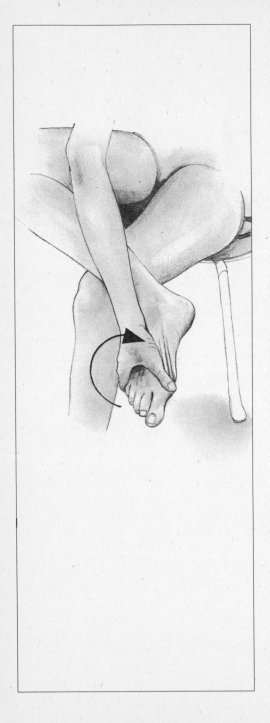

DIAGNOSTIC VERIFICATION

In looking for signs of this injury, you'll find that in walking each step usually hurts because it puts stress on the ligaments.

Test

To test for inner-ankle sprain, sit in a chair and cross your injured leg over your other one so that your injured ankle rests on the opposite knee. Relax your foot and grab hold of the front portion of your foot (top and bottom) with your hand, as shown. Now rotate the front of your foot with your hand, so that the big toe moves in a circular direction toward the floor. If you do this forcefully, it should cause discomfort in the strained ligament.

This injury can be confused with posterior tibialis tendinitis (p. 60) because this tendon passes behind and under the ankle bone and causes a similar pain when sprained.

TREATMENT CHOICES

Self-Treatment

You can treat this injury very effectively without medical help. All you need to do is buy an arch support at your drugstore and place it in your shoe. If it doesn't give you enough height and arch support to alleviate pain while you are walking, build it up where needed with some adhesive foam (also from the drugstore) until it is comfortable. If the support is properly constructed it should considerably reduce the pain you feel while walking—right away. It is important to wear this arch support continually for about three months. You *cannot* walk barefoot even for a short while. Each time you walk, a great deal of stress is placed on this ligament, and wearing the support takes the weight off the ligament. If you walk without the support, in slippers or barefoot before the ligament is fully healed, you can very easily retear the newly formed ligament fibers.

In addition, ice treatments can help speed your recovery. With luck and care you can resume moderate athletic activity after three or four weeks if you can do so without pain. After three months, you can begin to use your ankle without the support, but if there is any pain, use the support a little longer until you can wean yourself off of it.

Medical Treatment

1. DEEP MASSAGE OR DEEP FRICTIONING: This treatment can often aid in circulation and thereby help the fibers heal more quickly.
2. INJECTION: An injection of corticosteroid, when effective, can work within three to five days. However, injections are difficult because this treatment works only if *all* the sprained fibers are injected, and often fibers can be missed. In that case, pain will return. And even if injection treatments do work, you must wear your arch support for two to three weeks. If the ligament was badly sprained, the ligament fibers may have stretched and been lengthened. This stretching makes it vulnerable to reinjury. In these cases a proliferant injection to tighten and strengthen the ligament can be useful.
3. ORTHOTICS: If you have difficulty constructing your own arch support, you may wish to have a sports podiatrist make you one. He may choose to give you a pair of molded arch supports to change the position and alignment of both arches so that you feel balanced while walking.

Rehabilitation

See the five Foot, Ankle, Shin, and Calf exercises on pages 266–67.

Pain Under the Heel of the Foot
(Stoned Heel—Periostitis)

WHAT IS IT?

Probably this injury got its name because it feels as if you have a stone in the heel of your shoe. Stoned heel is in fact a bruise on the bottom of the heel of your foot which makes walking painful. It is actually the bone skin, or periosteum—a fluid-filled protective sheath that covers all bones—that is irritated and inflamed in this injury.

HOW AND WHY

I remember having this injury many times as an adolescent. I really loved to jump and frequently smashed my heel into the floor. This would lead to periodic hobbling around for three to four weeks.

In adults this injury usually occurs to runners whose heels strike the ground too severely or to any athletes who accidentally land on the heel with too much force. Sometimes the pain is felt right after you injure it, but more often you wake up the next morning unable to walk without pain, especially when barefooted. It feels like a bruised bone, but you rarely see a black-and-blue spot. Stoned heel is always caused by a trauma of some sort, and sometimes in addition to bruising the bone cover you also bruise the surrounding tissues under the heel.

DIAGNOSTIC VERIFICATION

This is one of those cases where just feeling the injured area is often enough. Press your fingers deeply into the bottom of your heel or try walking on your heels while barefoot. If you don't remember a traumatic incident and you haven't been active in sports lately, see your doctor to check for gout. Gout is a form of arthritis that may give you a strange pain in the heel or big toe for no apparent reason.

TREATMENT CHOICES

Self-Treatment

If you try a combination of rest, ice treatment, and cushioning—such as Dr. Scholl's Foam Cushioning—in your shoes, it should be effective within four to six weeks. Try not to walk too much, and never go barefoot. In addition, you can place adhesive foam or a heel cup in your shoes. Both of these can be purchased at a drugstore or a running-shoe store. Take care not to go back to activity too soon, as this injury is very likely to recur.

Medical Treatment

If you want to get better quickly, an injection of corticosteroid under the periosteum works in about a week.

Sharp Pain Through the Front of the Foot

(Interosseus Strain)

WHAT IS IT?

When you have sharp pain in the front part of the foot between one or several of the bony extensions of the toes, you are suffering from interosseus strain. It can be felt toward the top or bottom of the foot, or straight through the foot. This injury is a tearing of the muscle (A) that lies between the metatarsal bones of the foot. These muscles help to stabilize the front part of the foot. They prevent the toes from spreading apart when you walk and are called upon to work each time you take a step.

HOW AND WHY

This strain is frequently noticed when you get out of bed in the morning and are walking barefoot. A sharp pain is felt

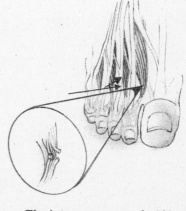

The interosseus muscle (A)

with each step. This may follow a day of heavy exertion, but not necessarily. When shoes are worn the pain is lessened or eliminated because the shoe is now stabilizing the front of the foot. In severe cases the pain persists during walking, shoes or no shoes. This knifelike pain is usually between the bones of the third and fourth toes. In mild cases, the pain may last for a few weeks, disappear for a short while, and return again with increased activity.

In this injury, small muscle tears frequently occur as a result of fatigue in the leg. The muscles of the leg tire and the brunt of the body's weight falls on these very weak and small muscles between the toes. They frequently tear in several places at once, and when they heal a matted scarring usually develops. It is this scar tissue that then retears under prolonged exertion.

DIAGNOSTIC VERIFICATION

Test
To test for interosseus strain clasp your hands underneath the ball of your foot just behind the toes and firmly exert pressure on both sides of your foot by squeezing your hands together. If you have this injury the squeezing will produce the pain. Diagnosis can be a little tricky because this injury can be confused with two others that we haven't covered in this book. One is inflammation of a nerve that runs between the toes, which is treated by injection into the nerve. The other is a small stress fracture of one of the bones of the foot (metatarsal), which requires rest to heal.

TREATMENT CHOICES

Self-Treatment
To treat yourself, wrap some tape securely around the metatarsal region to help hold it together. Be sure the tape doesn't bind you too much during walking. Two or three weeks' rest is often effective if the strain is not too severe. Try not to walk barefoot. If the pain tends to re-

cur, scar tissue is forming and you need some medical treatment.

Flex and point your toes many times throughout the day.

Medical Treatment
1. DEEP MASSAGE OR DEEP FRICTIONING: If the tearing is in the fibers near the skin surface, deep frictioning can be used to treat it. This area is very sensitive, however, and treatment can be extremely painful.
2. INJECTION: An injection of corticosteroid along the entire segment of the torn muscle is a very effective treatment.

7

The Knee

It is rare to go to a basketball game and not see at least one player with a knee wrapped up. The knee, the largest joint in your body, is often thought to be the place most vulnerable to athletic injuries. Many people who are actively involved in sports end up with some kind of knee injury, and on a given day in any locker room you can usually overhear a conversation about "my bum knee."

Why is the knee so vulnerable? Well, in part it's because the knee has less mobility than many other joints. Take your foot and ankle, for example. The ankle-and-foot mechanism can move forward and backward, and also has some side-to-side motion. Your knee simply moves forward and backward like a hinge and can tolerate only very limited amounts of side-to-side or twisting motion. Therefore, whenever falls, collisions, or weird accidents occur that twist or wrench the knee, you are almost bound to end up with some knee injury.

Another reason your knee is so vulnerable is that it is a very intricate and complex mechanism and many things can go wrong. We know of about twenty-five to thirty definite injuries to the knee, but in addition there are strange pains that appear and disappear in the knee that we know little about.

In the last decade jogging and running have gained tremendous popularity, and with this increase in runners there has been a large increase in knee injuries. Very few people have perfectly aligned knees, but the slight deviations of alignment that so many of us have usually cause no problems. Sometimes, however, these slight deviations add up to an injury if you get involved in activity that is stressful on the knees, such as running, basketball, or soccer.

Though the knee is complex, diagnosing knee injuries can be straightforward. The difficulty in diagnosis lies in the fact that people who have knee injuries often don't get to physicians who have expertise in this area. Often you can readily pinpoint the general location of your pain (e.g., in the front of your knee rather than the back) and in doing this you have already narrowed the possibilities down to four or five injuries. The exception is pain felt deep within the center of the knee. In these cases the cause of the injury is more elusive. Sometimes, although it's fairly rare, knee pain can be referred from hip and back injuries—that is, it is felt at a distance from the site of the injury (e.g., an irritation in the hip joint causing a generalized pain in the front of the knee).

The knee joint is made up of the joining of the thigh and shinbones with a small rounded bone in front called the patella or kneecap. The knee joint bends and straightens with a small twisting motion that isn't usually apparent. The bones of your knee are held together by strong cords called ligaments. Two are strategically placed to prevent the bones of the knee from moving side to side. There is a strong ligament cord at either side of the knee. The one on the inside (ligament A in the first illustration) prevents the knee from collapsing inward, and the outer one (ligament B in the first illustration) prevents the knee from col-

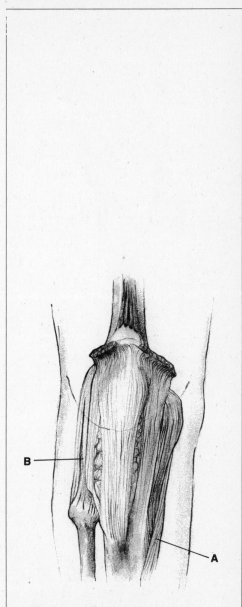

The knee, showing the medial collateral ligament (A) and the lateral collateral ligament (B)

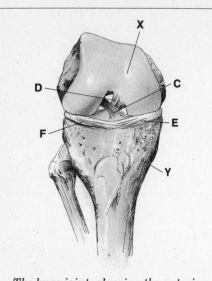

The knee joint, showing the anterior cruciate ligament (C), the posterior cruciate ligament (D), the medial coronary ligament (E), the lateral coronary ligament (F), the Teflon-like articular cartilage (X), and the tibia (Y)

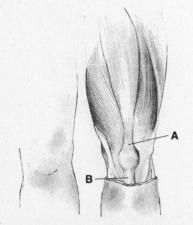

An injured patella tendon (A) and its lower portion—sometimes called the patella ligament (B)

lapsing outward. There are two ligaments (C and D in the second illustration) deep within the knee that prevent abnormal movement of the shinbone forward and backward.

Your knee has two types of cartilage. One is a thin, shiny, Teflon-like material (X), which coats the touching surfaces of all bones. This layer allows the bones to glide over one another easily. If this material wears away through a combination of misalignment and too much stress on the knee, it can cause long-standing arthritis in the knee, also called chondromalacia.

The other type of cartilage in the knee is the meniscus. Each knee has two of these smooth, shock-absorbing cartilages which are about a quarter-inch thick. They lie between the thigh bone and shinbone and are usually referred to colloquially as the knee cartilages. These cartilages are attached to the shinbone (or tibia, Y) by long, thin, circular ligaments (E and F).

Nicknames for the muscles that control the knee are the quads and hamstrings. The powerful quadriceps muscle of the front thigh is not one muscle but a group of four muscles working together. Just above the kneecap, they attach onto the patella tendon (A), which then envelops the kneecap, passing over it and attaching below to the shin bone. The lower portion of this tendon is alternatively referred to as the patella ligament (B) or the patella tendon—technically it is a tendon functioning as a ligament. (One difficulty with anatomy is that it's a lot like Russian novels: the same structure, or character, will often have two, three, or even four different names. In this case we will stick with patella tendon.) When the quadriceps muscles of the thigh contract, they pull on the patella tendon and cause the knee to straighten.

Now let's move to the hamstrings (*above right*)—the collective name for the three powerful muscles in the back of the thigh. The tendons of the hamstring muscles cross behind the knee joint and attach on either side of the knee (A and B). This muscle-tendon group bends the knee. I mention the hamstring tendons in this section because they often account for knee injuries in the back of the knee.

Another source of potential knee problems is found in the bursas. There are many bursas within the knee, and these fluid-filled sacs offer protection and cushioning. The ones most frequently injured in the knee are the ones beneath the kneecap. In the illustration, the bursa underneath the kneecap is shown as one continuous sac, but in actuality it has three sections that act independently. Each section has its own name, and usually they are injured separately.

You now have a picture of the basic structures of the knee.* With this information in mind, you are ready to find your specific injury. The first thing to do is to take a careful look at your knee and try to locate the general area of your pain. Now look at the illustration accompanying the "Locating Your Injury" section, and find the arrow or arrows that are closest to the location of your pain. From there go to the page numbers that are indicated. Once you have located the area of your pain, there will be only two or three injury descriptions to read through.

The picture becomes a little more complicated, but not impossible to understand, if there are several areas of pain. In these cases, find the location of the most painful area first and explore these injuries. Don't be surprised if two or more areas sound applicable because it's not uncommon to have more than one knee injury. A weakness caused by an injury to one part of the knee can cause the knee's alignment to be thrown off. This forces you to overstress other ligaments or tendons which may then become injured.

The last potential stumbling block is diffuse pain deep within the knee. If you are suffering from this type of pain, refer to the list of possibilities included in the diagram text.

LOCATING YOUR INJURY
Find the arrow in the drawing that corresponds approxi-

*I have omitted several small ligaments and tendons because they are rarely involved in knee injuries.

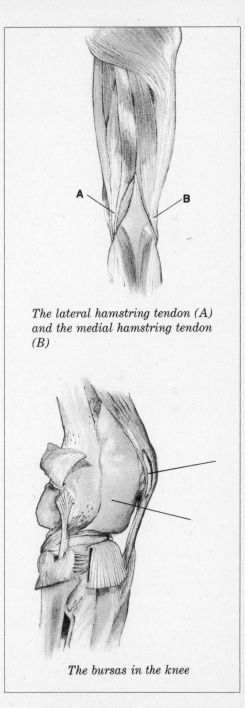

The lateral hamstring tendon (A) and the medial hamstring tendon (B)

The bursas in the knee

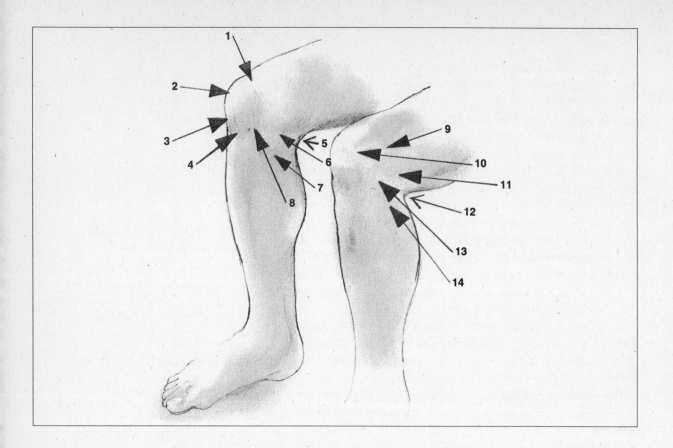

mately to where you feel pain. This list will guide you to the name and page number of your injury.

Be sure to read the entire Rehabilitation chapter before use of the rehabilitative exercises so that you can use them best.

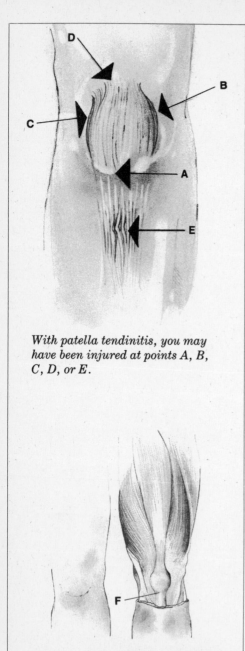

With patella tendinitis, you may have been injured at points A, B, C, D, or E.

Pain is most often felt at point F.

Pain in the Front of the Knee
(Patella Tendinitis)

WHAT IS IT?

The following is a story often heard by doctors and therapists treating knee injuries: "After I run for two or three miles my knee(s) begins to hurt. So I rest for a day or so and I feel fine. The next time I run the same thing happens." What's the problem? Something I've dubbed the most frequently misunderstood knee injury because it's been given at least four different names, and because the pain from this injury can be felt in many different areas, making it hard to evaluate. It actually is a strain and/or partial tearing of the patella tendon that crosses over the kneecap. The strain and/or tearing can occur above, below, or on the extreme inside or outside of the kneecap (A,B,C,D, or E). The pain is usually perceived as a generalized ache in the front of the knee just below the kneecap (F).

Most tendons serve only one muscle, but the patella tendon serves the four strong muscles that form the quadriceps at the front of the thigh. You can imagine that this is quite a load, but this tendon is one of the strongest and thickest tendons of the body. When the quadriceps contract they pull on the patella tendon, which in turn straightens the leg.

HOW AND WHY

This very common injury—variously called "runner's knee," "hiker's knee," "biker's knee," etc.—usually develops gradually and often comes and goes according to the amount of activity performed. Sometimes the pain starts several hours after a strenuous activity or even the following day. The pain is often felt when walking and especially when climbing stairs, but at times it hurts when walking downstairs as well. With this injury, doing deep-knee bends is frequently painful, particularly when straightening up. If your injury is recent and somewhat acute, it may ache all the time.

There are two types of patella tendinitis: recent and long-standing. In a recent injury, some of the fibers are actually torn apart. In a long-standing case, the fibers that were torn apart have healed poorly, forming a matted scar that is painful and tends to retear under each new strenuous exertion. A severe recent case, if left unattended, may become chronic.

There are several causes of patella tendinitis. The most common view is that the tendon tears because it is under too much stress. This can be caused by an improper warm-up, because a muscle that is not warmed up thoroughly remains stiff and somewhat rigid, thereby placing more stress on the tendon. Poor alignment is often at the root of the problem. If the foot turns out while the knee moves straight ahead during athletic activity, inordinate stress is placed on a small portion of the tendon and can cause the strain. Unless the alignment is corrected, the tendon will probably tear repeatedly.

Additionally, excess muscle tension in the thigh is a primary cause of patella tendinitis, because a tense muscle fatigues more quickly and causes strain to the tendon. Other contributing factors are poor form in your particular athletic activity and running and jumping on cement surfaces.

DIAGNOSTIC VERIFICATION

Diagnosing this injury can be tricky because the pain comes and goes. For the best results, try testing for this injury after an activity that makes your knee feel sore.

Test

While doing this test it's best to wear shoes. Stand facing the wall, about a foot away. Bend your injured knee and place your foot against the wall, as shown. Now push your lifted foot into the wall as hard as you can, as if you are trying to push the wall in. Does that cause you pain? If the

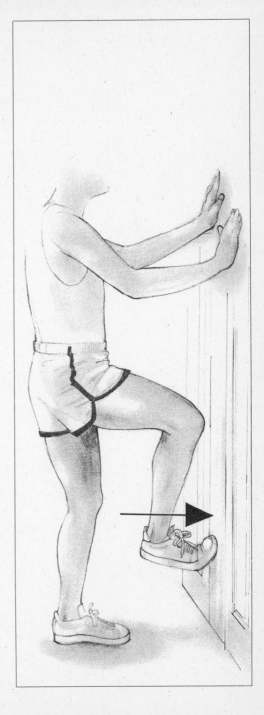

answer is yes, you have patella tendinitis.

Because the patella tendon is extremely powerful, testing it may sometimes be a problem. If you did the test above and didn't feel pain, it may be because you weren't able to put enough stress on the tendon to cause discomfort. Try going up and down a lot of stairs. You could try to stress the knee further with activity and test it again or seek out a qualified professional for help.

A further confusion is that this injury is often mistaken for chondromalacia (see p. 103) or bursitis of the knee, p. 130, where the pain is felt farther under the kneecap and the aching sensation is similar. On top of this, you can have more than one of these injuries at the same time. If you're confused you're not alone. Each injury must be treated separately to figure it out. It's usually too difficult to do by yourself, so seek some professional help if you have a mix of too many symptoms.

TREATMENT CHOICES

Self-Treatment

If you feel this type of pain, it's important to stop your activity immediately. If your injury is recent, you can apply the ice treatment along with the Knee Extension exercise on page 268. After a week or two of rest, you can begin some mild activity, such as easy jogging, to maintain the strength and integrity of the tendon. Don't push yourself too much. Only exercise as much as you can without feeling discomfort during or after the activity. Gradually increase your activity load and continue the ice treatment daily with bending and straightening of the knee. While moving your iced knee, be sure to straighten it fully to engage all the tendon fibers.

In general, if the tearing of the patella tendon is mild to moderate, rest and a little luck will result in proper healing. If you're not better in three or four weeks, or if your injury is an old one, you will probably need some of the medical help that follows.

Medical Treatment

1. DEEP FRICTIONING: Though very effective, this is a painful treatment.
2. INJECTION: The injection of corticosteroids is also beneficial. In fact, in certain difficult cases of long-standing injury, injections of corticosteroids are often the *only* effective treatment. One or two injections are usually all that is required.
3. ORTHOTICS: If poor foot alignment is the cause of your patella tendinitis, a molded arch support, accompanied by rest for a brief period, is often curative. The orthotic helps to redistribute the weight evenly.

Rehabilitation

See Knee Extension and Up, Out, In, Down exercises, pages 266, 267. Do them first without and then with weights.

Pain Deep Inside the Knee

(Cruciate Ligament Tears)

WHAT IS IT?

Though we discuss some injuries that are worse, this can be a serious, painful, and long-term injury. An aching pain is experienced deep inside the knee toward the front, toward the back, or all the way through the knee. It's hard to locate the exact spot of the pain because it is so deep inside.

There are two cruciate ligaments (C and D in the illustration); and you can strain or tear one or both of them. When football players injure these ligaments they are often ruptured completely in half. In less serious athletic injuries one ligament is usually sprained.

The cruciate ligaments crisscross diagonally deep inside the knee joint, and stabilize it in forward-to-backward movement. One ligament goes from the back of the thigh bone to the front of the shinbone and the other crosses

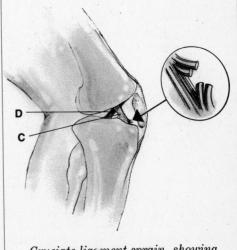

Cruciate ligament sprain, showing the anterior (C) and posterior (D) cruciate ligaments

from the front of the thigh bone to the back of the shin inside the knee joint.

HOW AND WHY

Usually it's a very weird athletic fall or accident that causes this sprain, although I have seen several tears occur during a sprint race. The injury often begins with a sharp pain at the back, or deep within the knee, followed by swelling and increased pain in a few hours. With time the pain becomes a dull ache rather than a sharp pain.

I remember a young runner who was injured during a British trial for the Olympic team. She was out in front in the middle of a hundred-meter race when she tripped, heard a snap, and was seized by a searing pain that forced her to stop and limp off the track. A physician quickly diagnosed it as being a sprained cruciate ligament.

This ligament can also be torn slowly, over a period of time, in any strenuous athletic activity that involves running, although this is not usually how it happens. In these cases, pain comes on gradually and is often felt only after a strenuous activity. In some cases, it can also be felt while squatting down to pick something up or when sitting cross-legged. There may be no swelling, but the leg may feel unstable or weak.

If there was no accident involved, these ligaments may have been torn for another reason: the muscles of the thigh were extremely tired and gave up their share of the load of supporting the leg. This placed more weight on the ligaments than they could absorb, resulting in fatigue and slow tearing. People who do a lot of yoga and sit for long periods of time in a lotus position can, over months, stretch and weaken the cruciate ligaments. They are then more vulnerable to this type of injury.

DIAGNOSTIC VERIFICATION

A word of caution: Only attempt these tests if your pain is mild; if your pain is severe, see a physician.

Test 1

Sit in a chair and bend your lower leg at a 90° angle. Grasp the back of your calf, just below the knee, and slide your foot back three or four inches, keeping only the ball of your foot on the floor, as shown. Now, forcefully press your lower leg forward with your hands. If this causes you discomfort, ligament C, the anterior cruciate, is torn.

There are two tests for the other ligament, D. For the second one (Test 3) you will need someone to help you.

Test 2

Lie down on the floor and place the back of your heel on a hard chair so that your thigh and calf form an approximate right angle. Now press your heel straight down into the

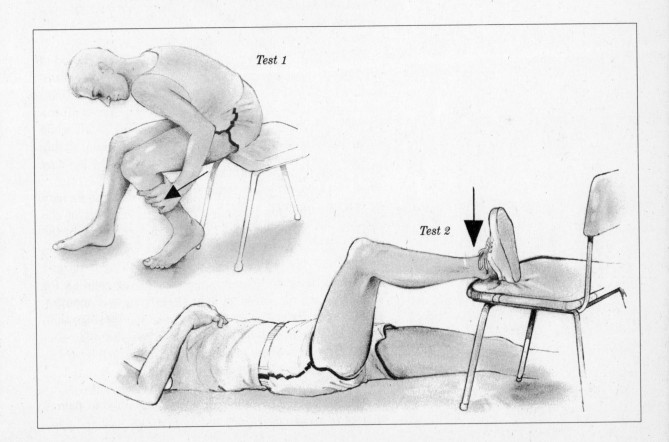

Test 1

Test 2

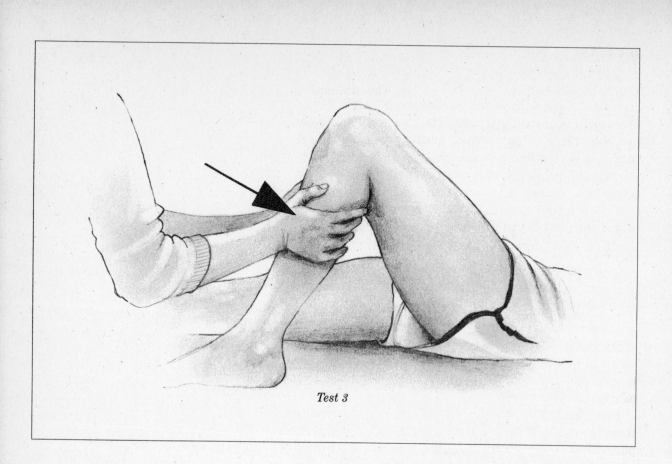

Test 3

chair toward the floor. If that causes pain deep inside your knee you have probably strained ligament (D), the posterior cruciate ligament. (If it causes pain in the back of your knee, it may be something different; see Hamstring Tear behind the knee, p. 99.)

Test 3

Lie on the floor and bend your injured knee, placing the sole of your foot on the ground slightly turned outward. Have a friend sit on your foot and take hold of your lower leg about four inches below your knee. As you relax your leg, your friend should push forward and down four or five times, forcefully. If that causes you discomfort it is ligament D (the posterior cruciate ligament) that is torn.

In mild cases, when the pain comes and goes, it is often helpful to stress the injury before testing it, by doing the activity that usually brings on your pain. This will enable the test to work better.

If while doing these tests you notice a lot of wobbly movement of the knee, one or both of the cruciate ligaments may be permanently stretched and lengthened. This adds to a feeling of instability in the knee and makes you prone to knee injury. Also see Water on the Knee, p. 113.

TREATMENT CHOICES

Self-Treatment

It is important to stress that this can be a painful, long-term, horrid injury. If you have swelling or severe pain or can't bend or straighten your leg fully, be sure to go to your doctor immediately. Even with a moderately severe strain you can expect a deep ache off and on in your knee for six to twelve months, and this is only if athletic activity is curtailed. If you don't take special care of yourself the pain can go on indefinitely.

There is little self-treatment that can be done because these ligaments are so deep in the knee. Ice treatment applied for six to eight hours a day with the Knee Extension exercise, p. 268, during the first five to seven days after the injury can reduce the initial pain so that you can walk more easily. At first you will want to limit your walking greatly. Athletic activities need to be resumed very slowly, and deep-knee bends will only cause trouble. In short, this injury takes a lot of patience.

Medical Treatment

1. SURGERY: In rare instances where the ligament is torn completely in half, surgery is the only treatment.
2. INJECTION: Where there is *not* a complete rupture, corticosteroid injection successfully speeds recovery if the correct spot is injected. A diagnostic injection of an anaesthetic to localize the exact spot is usually performed first.

    The young woman who strained a cruciate ligament during the British Olympic team trials was told she would be out for six to nine months with at least three months in a plaster cast. She then found a physician experienced in injecting these deep ligaments; within one week after a corticosteroid injection she was running again, and after three weeks she ran in another hundred-meter race, subsequently winning many sprint races.

An injection of proliferant is particularly helpful if the injury is recent or long-standing, or ranges from mild strain to a partial tear. It works slowly, to strengthen and tighten the ligament.

Since the ligament is so deep in the knee, it is difficult to administer the injection precisely, and many physicians will not attempt it. In some cases the ligament is permanently stretched in spite of injections, leaving the knee with a chronic feeling of instability and weakness. Some of this wobbliness can be overcome if you build up and maintain extremely strong thigh muscles.

Rehabilitation
See all of the Knee and Thigh exercises on pages 268–69.

Pain at the Outside of the Knee
*(Tendinitis of the Tensor Fascia Lata Tendon)**

WHAT IS IT?

This injury is new on the scene: it's been occurring more frequently with the gain in popularity of long-distance running. With this strain or tear of the tendon, the pain is felt at the outside of the knee (A) or at the outside of the thigh just above the knee (B).

The tensor fascia muscle is a short, strong muscle located at the upper portion of the outer thigh. This muscle is attached to the top of the shinbone just below the knee by a very long, strong, thick fascia that in this part of the

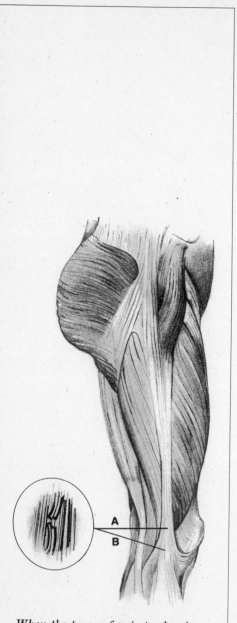

When the tensor fascia tendon is torn, you feel pain at (A) or (B).

*This is a strong fascia which functions as a tendon. It is also anatomically called the ilio-tibial tract.

body is functioning as a tendon. If you remember our earlier discussion of fascia, it's fascinating stuff because it has many functions and can take so many forms in the body. Here we will refer to it as a tendon.

HOW AND WHY

As mentioned above, this kind of tendinitis occurs most frequently in joggers or long-distance runners. It is a fatigue injury and can occur only if you push your body too far beyond its limit. The thigh muscles become tired and the knee gets a little wobbly. Extra stress is then placed on this tendon and injury occurs. Each time you run an aching pain usually returns more quickly than before. In some cases, pain occurs after you've run a certain number of miles. Although pain often subsides overnight, in severe cases it becomes painful to walk. With this injury there is never any swelling. Until the tendon is strong again, sports that require side-to-side movement, such as racquetball, basketball, and football, will tend to reinjure it.

DIAGNOSTIC VERIFICATION

Test

Stand with the outside of your injured leg up against a wall. Flex your foot, lifting the front of your foot an inch or two from the floor. Keeping your heel firmly in place, and with your leg straight, push the front outside of your foot into the wall with a great deal of force, as illustrated. This should reproduce your pain.

This injury is often confused with the more common lateral coronary ligament tear (p. 127) because the pain is often felt in the same area. If you have any doubts, do the test for lateral coronary ligament tear as well.

TREATMENT CHOICES

Self-Treatment

Ice treatment with the Side-Lying Lift, p. 269, done for

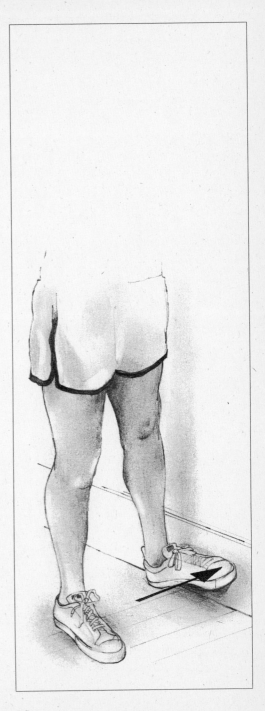

several weeks while limiting your activities to those that don't cause pain, is the most effective self-treatment. When you return to activity, swimming is probably the best thing to start for the first few weeks. If you feel pain-free for two weeks, begin running only very easy mileage that causes no pain.

Medical Treatment
1. DEEP FRICTIONING: This is an effective treatment for this injury. It should be accompanied by deep massage of the thigh to aid blood circulation.
2. INJECTION: Corticosteroid injection works well here if the strain does not cover a large area.

Rehabilitation
See all six Knee and Thigh exercises, pages 268–69.

Kneecap Dislocating to the Side
(Dislocating Patella)

WHAT IS IT?

When you dislocate your kneecap, it literally jumps out of its groove and moves to the outside of the knee, where it does not belong. Usually you can see it sitting there, but sometimes it goes back in place quickly—so quickly that you may not notice what happened. The pain can be so excruciating that at first you feel it everywhere. However, it usually concentrates at the front and outside of the knee.

The kneecap, or patella, sits between the thigh and shin bones; it's triangular in shape and slides in a groove provided by nature in the front and bottom of the thigh bone. The patella protects the knee joint and acts as a fulcrum (like the bar in a see-saw) for the tendon that passes over it. This mechanism increases the strength efficiency of the front thigh muscles by about 40 percent.

HOW AND WHY

Children, especially those between the ages of eight and
thirteen, are the most common victims of dislocating knee-
caps. Although the condition is sometimes outgrown, it often persists in young athletes and adults. It usually
happens during a running activity, but it can occur when
you make a sharp turn while walking. The kneecap moves
out of its groove, over to the side. There is a sharp pain,
the leg locks in a bent position, and usually you fall down.
Youngsters soon learn to treat themselves by forcefully
straightening the leg, or correcting it by popping the
kneecap back into place with their hands. Both of these
methods are often accompanied by a loud *click*. Then, feeling fine, they usually resume their activity. However, after a short period of time, the knee often swells and hurts
for several days.

Dislocations occur in some individuals because their patella is either too small for the groove in the thigh bone or
it is not as firmly anchored as it should be by the tendon
that passes over it. It is therefore liable to slide out of its
track when the knee is in certain positions and under
stress.

When this problem continues into late adolescence and
adulthood it often makes you afraid to be athletically active.

DIAGNOSTIC VERIFICATION

This injury is sometimes confused with a torn cartilage
(p. 106), because some of the symptoms are the same.
There is one simple test, shown on the next page, that
usually confirms the diagnosis.

Test

Sit on the floor with your leg straight but relaxed. Place
your thumb on the inside edge of your kneecap as shown
and gently push the kneecap toward the outside (in the direction of the dislocation). You should be able to move it
quite far.

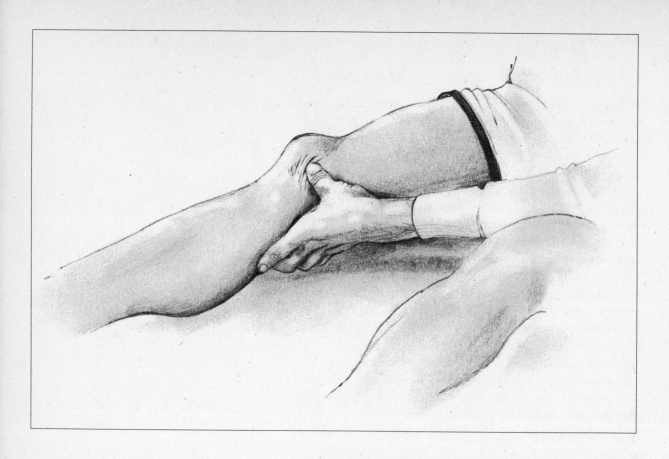

If you have a dislocating patella you will *automatically* stop the movement by a sudden contraction of the muscles of the thigh, which will pull the patella back into place. This happens involuntarily when you reach a place that feels "too far." Just reading this or thinking about it will usually cause a fear reaction if you have this problem.

TREATMENT CHOICES

Self-Treatment
When this problem occurs in children it is often outgrown as the patella grows in size, making the fit better and helping the muscles to strengthen. When the kneecap dislocates, the leg should immediately be forcefully straightened. The longer it is left in a dislocated position, the more pain and inflammation follow.

Ice and rest do no good as a cure, but the passage of time often takes care of the condition.

Quadriceps exercises (pp. 268-69, the first three) to build up the front thigh muscles often keep the injury under control so that the dislocation will happen only infrequently. Straightening the knee with weights on the foot is the best exercise for this problem.

Medical Treatment
Surgery is usually recommended in extreme cases. It is only sometimes effective. Consult several doctors for their opinions.

Pain at the Back, Outside, or Inside of the Knee
(Hamstring Tendon Tear Near the Hamstring Attachment at the Knee)

WHAT IS IT?

This isn't exactly a knee injury, but it often masquerades as one. Hamstring strains usually occur in the mid- or upper thigh (p. 185). But sometimes the lower tendons become inflamed and painful. If you are sitting in a chair you can easily feel those stringlike tendons as they pass behind the knee at the extreme inner and outer edges. When you hurt them, you feel pain in several places, depending on where this tendon is strained. Pain can be felt behind the knee at the inside (A in the illustration) or the outside (B). Or it can be felt at the hamstring attachments that are in front of and below the knee (C and D).

All three hamstring muscles begin at the bottom of the pelvis (E) and originate from one common tendon at the top of the back thigh. Then they spread out into separate muscles. One of these muscles is on the outside of the thigh (F) and passes over the back, outside portion of the knee. Its tendon attaches below the knee on the outside of the lower leg (C). The other two muscles (G and H) over-

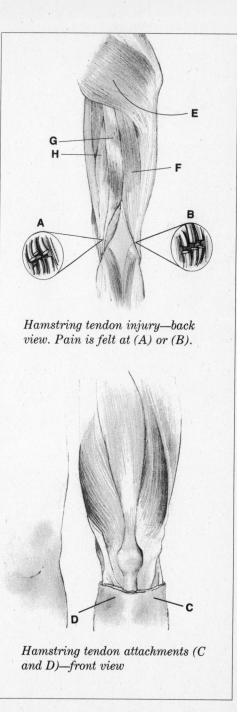

Hamstring tendon injury—back view. Pain is felt at (A) or (B).

Hamstring tendon attachments (C and D)—front view

lap each other so only one is readily seen. They progress gradually inward toward the inside of the back thigh, crossing the back of the knee joint toward the inside, attaching to the shinbone just below the knee (D).

When these tendons are strained (A, B, C, or D) behind or just below the knee, the pain is often mistakenly diagnosed as coming from a knee injury, when in fact it is the hamstrings that are injured.

HOW AND WHY

Fatigue is the clearest cause of many hamstring tendon injuries. You push yourself beyond your limit and something gives. Sometimes there is a snapping sound and a searing pain is immediately felt. But more often the pain creeps up on you slowly after several days of intense physical activity or stretching. If it's minor, only running or jumping activities will cause pain, but if the injury is more severe, you'll feel pain even when walking.

People often wonder why this injury doesn't hurt as much or at all when they are all warmed up and at the height of an activity, but a few hours after they have stopped the activity they feel their pain again. This happens because you don't feel pain when tendons are warmed and their circulation is increased. However, as the circulation slows and the tendon cools, you begin to feel pain again.

Poor stretching technique,* or stretching done without a prior warm-up, is often a contributing factor to this tendinitis. Once you've injured a hamstring tendon, continued stretching can prevent the tendon from recovering. The stretching keeps tearing the newly formed delicate tissue. I've heard many people say they have been told that in order to get better they need to stretch their hamstring every day, and they are really frustrated to find after eight months that they are still in pain. In fact, it's the stretching that's keeping them from healing.

*See pp. 279–81 for elaboration of good and poor stretching techniques.

In order for your leg to function properly, there has to be a balanced ratio between your front-thigh and back-thigh muscles. This strength ratio is usually sixty to forty respectively. If you do exercises that work one set of muscles to the exclusion of the others, you unbalance the ratio and make yourself more vulnerable to hamstring injuries. Chronic excess tension in your thighs could also contribute to this tendinitis.

DIAGNOSTIC VERIFICATION

There are two tests for this injury. At least one of them should help you confirm your diagnosis.

Test 1
Lie on your back on the floor and place your heel on a chair

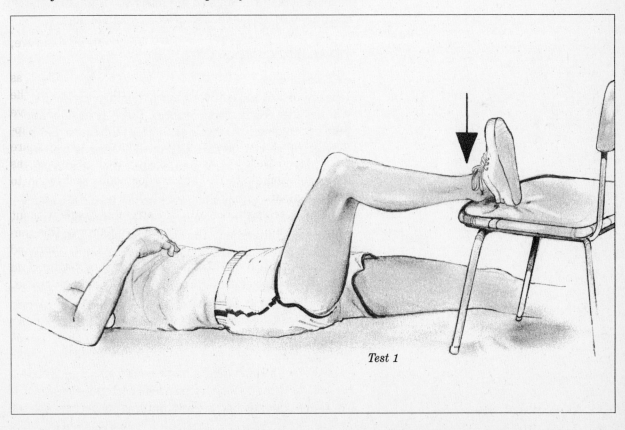

Test 1

with your leg bent at about a right angle. Press your heel straight down toward the floor forcefully, engaging your hamstring muscle. If you have a hamstring tear near the knee, it will hurt behind the knee or below the knee in the front. The semisharp pain you experience should be felt somewhere near the surface, *not* deep inside the knee. If you feel pain within the knee, it may be a deep ligament tear (cruciate ligament, p. 89).

Test 2

This test—which is slightly less reliable because it involves more structures—stretches the hamstring gently. The test will re-create your pain, whereas the previous test may not do so if the tendon strain is very slight. In a standing position, place the foot of your injured leg up on a chair. Keeping the injured leg fairly straight, stretch forward toward your knee. Stop when you feel pain.

TREATMENT CHOICES

Self-Treatment

It is important to keep your hamstring moving so that unwanted scar tissue does not form. But it is equally important not to do any exercise activities that cause you pain. Stretching should be curtailed until healing is well under way; only then can very gentle stretching be started if it does not cause pain. A good exercise to help you avoid scar-tissue formation while recovering from this injury is to bend and straighten your leg fully ten or fifteen times repeatedly throughout the day. You should work out a complete warm-up program before you re-enter activity. I have set out such a program in my book *Sports Without Pain*. Your recovery will be greatly enhanced if you use the ice treatment as often as possible. If you begin strenuous activity too soon and feel some discomfort, stop immediately and be patient for another several days before trying again.

If rest with some gentle movement doesn't get you better within three to four weeks, seek some medical help. If you keep reinjuring yourself, internal scar tissue often forms, weakening the tendon structure. This can be prevented with a brief period of friction treatment. Long-standing cases need to be treated by injection.

Medical Treatment
1. DEEP MASSAGE: This is often an effective treatment. The tendon and back thigh should be worked five or six times over a two-week period.
2. DEEP FRICTIONING: This procedure, although somewhat painful, works well. The tendinitis is a little more stubborn when the tear occurs right at the attachment to the bone, and in this case may require more treatments; but usually two to three weeks of treatment three times a week is sufficient.
3. INJECTION: Corticosteroid injections are also very effective in both the early and chronic stages, but should be combined with deep frictioning and adequate rehabilitation to ensure recovery.

Rehabilitation
See Hamstring Strengtheners, p. 269.

Pain Under the Kneecap
(Chondromalacia—Osteoarthritis of the Knee)

WHAT IS IT?

In recent years, chondromalacia has become the catchall term for knee injuries when specific knowledge is lacking. Patients often come in claiming they have chondromalacia, but in three out of every four cases they have something else.

The pain in true chondromalacia is usually a dull aching, felt very clearly under the kneecap. In severe cases the pain is felt to be more widespread.

Chondromalacia actually is the softening and thinning of cartilage. The undersurface of the kneecap (A) and the lower end of the thigh bone (B) which glides against the kneecap are both gliding surfaces covered with cartilage.

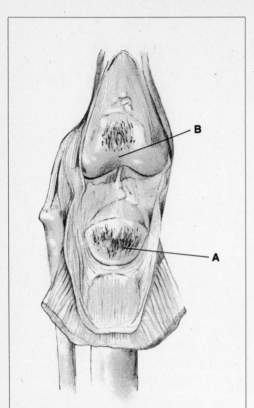

With chondromalacia, the undersurface of the kneecap (A) grinds against the thigh bone or femur (B).

For reasons that are often unknown, the cartilage softens and wears away on either or both of the contacting surfaces. In the accompanying illustration you are looking at the under surface of the kneecap (A), which for the purposes of illustration has been shown as pulled up and off of the thigh bone (B). The dark lines indicate the erosion of the cartilage on both of the contacting surfaces. When chondromalacia is painful, cartilage is probably markedly worn away in places and bone is grinding against bone. It almost always occurs in both knees simultaneously.

HOW AND WHY?

Chondromalacia is a lot like a hinge that is beginning to erode and needs oil. At first the knee creaks and grinds very faintly—you hardly pay it any mind. But with time and use the wearing away accelerates and the grinding sound becomes more noticeable. This injury usually does not occur in people who are not athletic. In normal wear and tear on the knee, the erosion of cartilage may take thirty years to happen or may not happen at all.

Your first signs of discomfort are usually mild aching during or after exercise, especially running or jogging. It gradually worsens over the next several months and you will have "good days" and "bad days," depending on how active you've been. As the cartilage wears you will find that you feel some pain walking uphill or upstairs, but the greater discomfort will occur when you walk downstairs, walk downhill, or kneel. In some cases, sitting with bent knees makes you ache, and in the most severe cases even walking is difficult.

Misalignment of the knee and foot is usually the prime cause of chondromalacia. For example, if the arches drop, making the feet pronate, the bone alignment within the knee joint is thrown out of balance. When your leg is misaligned, even in slight ways that normally aren't noticed, and you add the extra stress of a running sport, the stress on the knee and the consequent erosion are increased.

Another cause of chondromalacia can be a loose piece of

bone or cartilage floating in the joint space. It's as if a stray piece of metal became lodged in a finely meshed set of gears, destroying the smooth interlocking of the surfaces.

DIAGNOSTIC VERIFICATION

Test yourself if possible when you are feeling some discomfort.

Test
Do a deep-knee bend in a quiet room and listen for a grinding sound coming from your knee(s). This may or may not be painful.

Then sit on the floor and place the palm of your hand directly on your kneecap. Press down firmly and move your kneecap from side to side as far as you possibly can. Be sure to maintain the downward pressure of your hand. If you have chondromalacia this will cause a grinding feeling and pain, provided that you have the courage to press hard enough.

Some people have had grinding and cracking knees for years without pain. These individuals may have an extra-thick cartilage covering on the ends of their bones. When they later develop pain along with this grinding they assume they have developed chondromalacia. However, it is important to remember that this injury can be easily confused with patella tendinitis or bursitis of the knee, so if you have any doubts or questions, refer to those sections as well.

TREATMENT CHOICES

Self-Treatment
If you in fact have chondromalacia, there is relatively little you can do for yourself. If your pain goes away within a few weeks with quadriceps exercises or other self-treatments, you probably had something other than chondromalacia. The only effective thing you can do for yourself if you have this injury is to limit your activities to those that don't cause you pain.

Medical Treatment

1. ORTHOTICS: Orthotics are often an effective treatment (see p. 38) in the early stages: they place the bones of the feet in proper alignment and center the knee over the foot. This diminishes the pressure of abnormal rubbing between the two cartilage surfaces in the knee. If nothing else, orthotics often prevent a worsening of this condition.

2. INJECTION: DMPSO* has been used successfully since 1967 in treating chondromalacia in Europe. DMPSO is a thick, sterile solution which is injected into the joint and stays there permanently. It stops the pain by both lubricating the contacting bony surfaces and holding them apart.

   This treatment is not available at present in the U.S., although thousands have been treated with it successfully elsewhere. I mention this treatment here in the hope that it will be available in the near future.

   Proliferant injections are often helpful in cases that are not extremely severe.

Rehabilitation

Many claim that exercise is helpful, but I have personally never seen it as an effective, lasting treatment.

Torn Cartilage in the Knee

(Torn Meniscus)

WHAT IS IT?

Many an injury time-out on a football field signals another torn cartilage. This common and painful injury plagues many athletes and dancers. When the shock-absorbing cartilages (A and B) tear within the knee, pain is felt deep inside the knee. The pain, though deep in the knee, will be

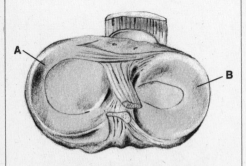

The knee cartilages—the lateral meniscus (A) and the medial meniscus (B)

*Dimethylpolysiloxane—not to be confused with DMSO.

either on the inside or the outside, depending on which cartilage is damaged.

The knee cartilages, or menisci, act as shock absorbers to facilitate and cushion the movement between your thigh bone and shinbone. They are shaped like half-moons and are slightly elastic. As you bend and straighten your knee, the cartilages slide slightly forward and backward within the knee. The menisci are attached by thin, long ligaments (the coronary ligaments) to the top of the shinbone and to the bottom of the thigh.

There are different types of cartilage tears. There can be a lengthwise tear (B-1 in the drawing); there can be a horizontal tear (B-2)—in this case a piece can actually

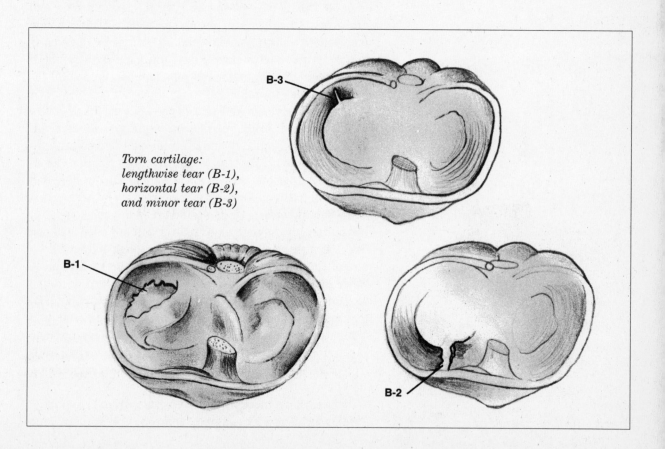

Torn cartilage: lengthwise tear (B-1), horizontal tear (B-2), and minor tear (B-3)

break off and float in the joint; and there can be minor tears such as B-3, which can also be very painful.

HOW AND WHY

This very common knee injury comes in two varieties—either mildly troublesome or severely debilitating, that is, horrible. Let's start with the slight tears. Your knee feels a little weak, there is frequently a slight clicking sound when you bend and straighten your knee, and occasionally when you accidentally twist your knee too much it feels like your leg is going to collapse under you . . . sometimes it actually does. Then you find yourself sitting on the floor with a bent knee that won't straighten and it hurts like the devil. If this is old hat to you, you jiggle your knee and straighten it and you can get up and walk. If this is a new experience, you may hobble home, call your doctor, or anxiously wait a few hours or days until you can straighten your knee. Often your knee swells and can be painful for up to a couple of weeks.

When you have a major tear of the knee cartilage you're always worried. Your knee is consistently weak and vulnerable and it regularly and unpredictably gives way under you, frequently getting stuck in a bent position. Even when it's not locking on you it's often painful, swollen, and a drag. A frequent fantasy is that you wish there was a spare-parts shop where you could trade in your knee.

Whether you have a minor tear or a major one, the knee locks because a piece of the torn cartilage moves into a part of the joint where there is no space for it. The piece either moves toward the center of the joint (B-1) or it flips over on itself, creating a thick double layer of cartilage (B-2) stopping the movement of the joint. It is impossible to straighten the leg without crushing the cartilage further. The muscles of the thigh contract as a reflexive, self-protective mechanism to prevent you from straightening the knee.

Torn cartilage most frequently results from a traumatic athletic accident. For example, someone crashes into your leg from the side in a football game; or you experience a bad fall in skiing, your bindings don't give quickly enough, and your knee is so painfully twisted that it takes the ski patrol to move you.

A less traumatic way to get injured is forced snap kicking in karate or standing up quickly after being in a squatting position for a long time the way you are when you're gardening.

In both of the less traumatic injuries above, your cartilage does not have enough time to slide into place and it gets partially crushed between the thigh bone and shinbone. When you tear your cartilage you usually injure one or two ligaments with it (see pp. 116, 125, and 127). In general, the inner side of your knee is more susceptible to injury, and if the pain is toward the inner side of your knee you have damaged the inner (medial) cartilage. If your pain is toward the outer side then you have injured the outer (lateral) cartilage.

DIAGNOSTIC VERIFICATION

The major diagnostic key in this injury is having your knee periodically buckle and lock. If this major symptom is missing it is difficult to know if you have a torn cartilage without one of the medical tests described below. Another important symptom is that your knee is painful deep inside—not only near the surface—and you are hesitant to straighten your knee all the way.

Orthopedic surgeons use one of two reliable diagnostic techniques. One is an arthrogram, in which an X ray is taken of the knee joint after dye has been injected into it. The dye then outlines the cartilage. The second procedure, arthroscopy, involves inserting an amazing tool that resembles a needle into the knee joint. This miniature microscope allows the doctor to observe most parts of the cartilage directly.

Frequently, the coronary ligament (p. 125 or p. 127) *rather than* the knee cartilage is torn, or the cartilage tear is properly diagnosed but the coronary ligament tear is missed and your pain may continue even after surgery. Also see Water on the Knee, p. 113.

Also see Water on the Knee, p. 113.

TREATMENT CHOICES

Self-Treatment

If you have a minor cartilage tear and your knee locks on you only occasionally, you may just need to learn how to unlock it quickly as many athletes have. It's helpful to find a doctor, therapist, or trainer to teach you how to unlock your knee. If you know how to unlock your knee quickly, the knee will not swell and will not be painful for more than a short while, if at all.

If you don't know how to manipulate your knee back into place, or if it's severely painful and swollen, be sure to get to a doctor quickly.

If this injury occurs to a minor degree—only every few months, say—you may choose to live with it rather than undergo surgery. However, if you make this decision, you may need to curtail certain kinds of activity that tend to bring it on.

Medical Treatment

1. INJECTION: In slight tears at the edge of the carti-lage—where it attaches to the ligament—some doc-tors will inject a mixture of dextrose lidocaine,* and corticosteroid, which can help control an acute in-flammation and then stimulate a self-healing cycle.

2. SURGERY: If the cartilage is torn badly and the pain and trouble are just too much, surgery is often a suc-cessful treatment. Cartilage has a very meager blood supply; therefore it rarely heals by itself and surgery is often your only choice. There is a greatly improved form of surgery that can be totally performed through a needle inserted into the side of the knee. With this surgical procedure, recovery time is three to four weeks rather than the three to four months required by more conventional procedures.

*A proliferant.

Rehabilitation
See all Knee and Thigh exercises, pp. 268–69.

Occasional Sharp Pain Within the Knee

(Loose Body in the Knee Joint)

WHAT IS IT?

You are walking along and *bang*—you get a sharp pain in your knee for no reason. You have a "loose body" injury—which is *not* the result of being overly relaxed. A "loose body" is actually a small fragment (A in the illustration) of bone or cartilage that has chipped off and is floating within a joint. Pain is felt deep within the knee when the loose fragment blocks the joint from certain movements.

HOW AND WHY

The pain from a loose body strikes without warning and is felt as a sharp twinge. It can happen as easily in athletic activity as in walking. The pain usually occurs when the knee is straight (though it occasionally occurs when the knee is bent) and weight is placed on the leg. The dislodged fragment gets stuck and crushed between the two bones. Along with the pain the knee sometimes locks in a straight position, causing you to fall—people with a loose body are usually very cautious about walking downstairs, because they know if the knee locks and then gives way they can suffer a serious accident.

Often only a shake of the leg is necessary to dislodge the loose body and walk again, but there is usually pain and swelling as the day progresses. The swelling subsides over the next few days or few weeks, depending on how irritated your knee gets. This injury is tricky because it has no consistent pattern and can return weekly, monthly, or even yearly. Sometimes a small loose body lodges in an

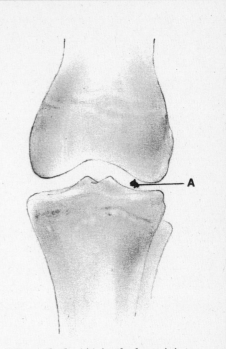

Loose body (A) in the knee joint

area of the knee joint where there is enough room for it to lie peacefully, so it rarely causes pain. Other times it's frequently in the wrong place at the wrong time. In some cases there are even several loose bodies found in the same knee joint.

The direct cause of this chipped piece of bone or cartilage is often unknown. It can occur as a result of a fall in which a piece of bone or cartilage is broken off. Where there is arthritis in the knee (chondromalacia), the bones rub against one another, and sometimes this slow erosion and wearing away of bone may result in small chips.

DIAGNOSTIC VERIFICATION

If the loose body is a fragment of cartilage, an X ray can't detect it because X rays only pick up bone. If it's a bone fragment, it is often very small and special detailed X rays called tomograms are necessary. In some cases, a procedure called an arthroscope or arthrogram done by a physician will confirm the presence of a loose body, but if the loose body is especially small it will miss it. The best way to evaluate this injury is through an understanding of where, how, and when you feel the pain.

TREATMENT CHOICES

Self-Treatment
Unfortunately, there is no known method of self-treatment for loose bodies. If there are certain activities that bring it on, you can, of course, avoid them. However, outside help is usually required to deal with this injury.

Medical Treatment
1. MANIPULATION: If the loose body gets stuck in the joint with some frequency, a special manipulation (described by Dr. James Cyriax*) can be used to move the piece to a different part of the joint where it may

*Cyriax and Russell, *Textbook of Orthopaedic Medicine*, vol. II (Baltimore, 1978), pp. 394, 398.

cause less trouble. This may have to be repeated three or four different times over a period of a week or two before it is successful. At best, of course, this is only a stop-gap measure.

2. KNEE WASH: This method of treatment has had a fair amount of success with small loose bodies. One needle is inserted on either side of the knee joint and a salt-water solution is flushed through the joint under pressure, driving the water and the loose piece out through the needle on the other side.

3. SURGERY: This procedure is often recommended to remove a loose body in a fairly young person. When young people have a loose piece made of bone, the nutrients within the knee joint will cause it to calcify (get larger over time) inside the joint. Leaving it in causes a reaction similar to having a stone grinding between the bones; it causes progressive deterioration and erosion of the joint.

   If the loose body is made of cartilage it is often very difficult to locate its exact position. Surgeons are therefore wisely hesitant about operating if they have to search around. Arthroscopy, surgery performed through a needle inserted in the knee rather than opening the knee, can be effective for loose-body removal and is much less disabling than regular surgery.

Water on the Knee / Swollen Knee
(Traumatic Arthritis or Inflammation)

WHAT IS IT?

This injury is rarely a loner. It usually tags along with injuries such as torn ligaments and torn cartilages. However, occasionally it makes a solo appearance.

Water on the knee is an irritation to the lining of the knee joint. This lining is a very thin membrane called the synovial membrane, which produces a small amount of fluid that lubricates the joint. When the lining gets irritated it overproduces fluid, which cuts down your movement and causes pain.

HOW AND WHY

When water on the knee is not a tagalong problem from a more serious injury it usually occurs through a fall or a jolt. The soccer player gets it by jamming his heel or foot directly down into the ground with a straight leg to stop the ball; the basketball player through a collision that's not severe enough to break a bone or injure a ligament. The knee swells over the next two to six hours and becomes warm, red, and painful throughout. What happens is that the fluid-producing membrane inside the joint goes haywire from the shock and overproduces fluid to bathe the concussed joint. It can produce more than eight ounces of liquid, which in turn causes tremendous pressure in the knee.

As mentioned above, water on the knee usually occurs with another injury. Almost all knee-ligament tears, torn cartilage, and loose-body problems produce swelling. In these cases the "water on the knee" usually disappears when the primary injury is taken care of. In some cases a swollen knee persists after the primary injury has healed and the treatment described below is then helpful.

If the swelling occurred without any obvious trauma or accident, it may be a symptom of a type of arthritis. If the swelling comes and goes, and you feel it in both knees or other joints, you should see a rheumatologist.

DIAGNOSTIC VERIFICATION

If your knee is blown up like a balloon you can't miss it; but if there is a small amount of swelling you might not notice it. If you have a diffuse knee pain whose cause is uncertain, compare both knees meticulously. If water on the knee is the primary problem your pain will be general rather than in a specific spot. Remember, if it is *specifical-*

ly located, check the ligament injuries in the later sections.

First, compare the heat of your knees by placing the back of your hand on one knee and then on the other. Is the injured knee hotter? If it's hot, it's swollen and inflamed. Now look carefully to see if the injured knee is red in comparison to your other knee.

Test 1

Lie down on your back and, grasping the ankle with both hands, pull first one heel and then the other toward your buttock. With a normal knee, you should be able to touch your buttock with your heel. If one leg is more limited or painful, it indicates swelling; if you can't do so, but both legs are limited equally, it's probably just the way you're built.

Test 2

Now stand up, put your foot on a chair, and press down above your knee (as illustrated) so that you straighten your leg with some force. If that is painful or you can't do it, there is probably extra fluid in your knee joint. When traumatic inflammation is present, you generally have a lot of trouble bending your knee and only a little bit of difficulty straightening it. Remember there may be pain in this test, or only a feeling of fullness that prevents you from completing the movement.

These same symptoms may be present in various kinds of arthritis. So if there was no accident, see your doctor about it.

TREATMENT CHOICES

Self-Treatment

If there is no single point of pain, apply ice treatment to the whole knee and avoid deep-knee bends, straightening your leg forcefully, or jarring movements such as running. Rest the knee for a while and see if the swelling subsides. This may take as long as three or four months. If the swelling is severe, it is of course better to see a doctor.

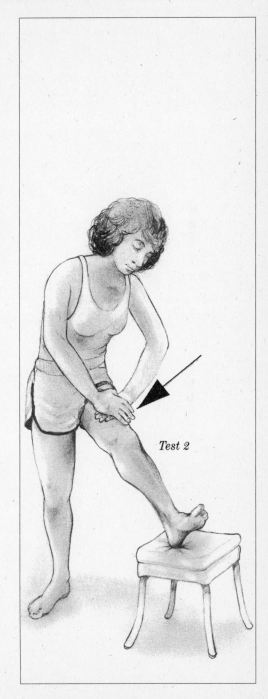

Test 2

Medical Treatment

The only method found effective for this injury is an injection of corticosteroid into the joint. One, or at most two, injections are all that is required. The pain and limitation of your movement should be gone within two or three days. However, if a ligament or other primary injury has been missed, the swelling will keep coming back. Be sure not to aggravate the joint for several weeks and be careful to move slowly back into full activity.

Pain at the Inner Side of the Knee
(Medial Collateral Ligament Tear)

WHAT IS IT?

This is *the* knee injury; more people suffer from this one than from any other. With this ligament sprain, some of the fibers have torn either in the middle (A in the illustrations) or near one of the ends (B and C). Regardless of where the fiber is torn, pain is felt directly on the inner side of the knee. This is the injury that usually prompts the phrase "my bum knee," for it has a habit of appearing and disappearing mysteriously.

There are three types of sprains you can have here: a mild sprain, where only a few fibers are damaged; a moderately severe sprain, where many fibers are torn; and an extremely severe one, where the ligaments tear completely in half.

This ligament is so important because it holds your leg together by connecting your thigh bone and shinbone at the inner side. It prevents the knee from buckling inward and keeps it on the track of forward-back movement.

HOW AND WHY

Suddenly, as if you had been hit by lightning, you find yourself on the ground. You were tackled or fell and your knee buckled inward. Perhaps you heard a snapping

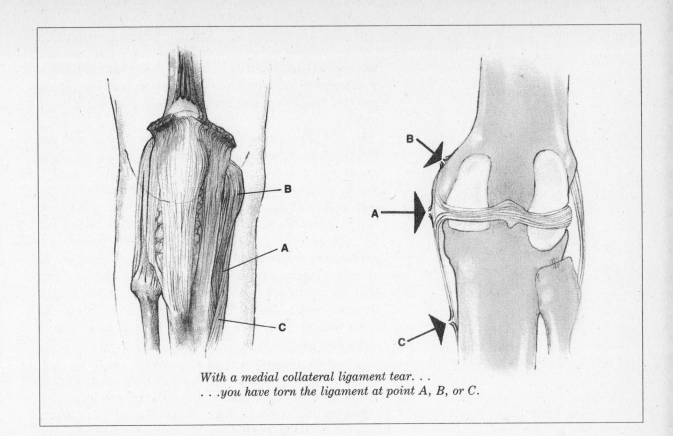

With a medial collateral ligament tear. . .
. . .you have torn the ligament at point A, B, or C.

sound, but more likely you missed it in the confusion of
your fall. Your knee hurts everywhere, and you hobble off
trying not to bend it. Over the next few hours the knee
swells, feels hot to the touch, and continues to ache. With
the passing hours, the knee stiffens, making bending and
straightening it difficult, and by the next day the pain begins to concentrate on the inner side of the knee. Your activity automatically becomes limited because walking is
painful and anything more strenuous is impossible.

Or you can be enjoying your daily exercise of tennis,
running, or racquetball, when you start feeling a twinge of
pain now and then. After a few weeks the pain settles on
the inside of your knee and is more constant. There may
be slight swelling or maybe not. You begin to notice pain
as you start playing; then it goes away; and an hour or so

after you're finished it hurts again. Your pain mysteriously disappears in the middle because the ligament gets so warmed up. Eventually you can no longer play without pain.

In both these cases the problem is the same: a torn medial collateral ligament. This mysterious injury has many personalities. It can come on quickly and be mild, moderate, or severe. Or it can come more slowly, like a building rain, and be either mild or moderately painful. No matter how it starts it often lingers for a long time or baffles you by coming and going. When your injury results from trauma it's easy to understand what caused it. When it comes on slowly the causes are subtle and often interlocking: poor leg alignment with turned-in knees, excess muscle tension—which leads to early fatigue—or loose or stretched-out ligaments caused by old sprains or poor stretching exercises.

A further complication of torn medial collateral ligaments is the "bum-knee" syndrome. In one way or another you've sprained your ligament, and though you have brief reprieves and begin to think you've beaten the problem, the pain mysteriously returns. It can recur with what you thought was a simple activity, such as helping a friend move some boxes up a flight of stairs, squatting for five minutes while you do a quick weeding of a garden, running a mile a day for two weeks, or making a block-long dash to catch the bus. Troublesome scar tissue that keeps retearing is the key to understanding this mystery. When your knee bends and straightens naturally this ligament moves freely across the bone. If it's injured and heals properly the scar tissue that's formed within the ligament does not interfere with this free movement. However, if your injury doesn't heal well, scar tissue may form between the ligament and the bone where it's not supposed to be. This scar tissue acts like a glue adhering the ligament to the bone so its free-sliding movement is more limited. If your activities are more strenuous and jarring, or involve twisting, the scar tissue does not hold and tears away from the bone. An hour or so later, when your ligament has cooled down, your pain returns. This cycle of poor healing and scar tissue retearing can happen hundreds of times over many years.

Given all its possibilities, it's easy to see why this is such a troublesome injury. We've covered its mild-to-moderate forms; in its most extreme form the ligament completely tears in half and your knee becomes so unstable that your immediate reaction should be to see a doctor.

DIAGNOSTIC VERIFICATION

One of the clearest diagnostic signs of this injury is the location of your pain. It's always on the inner side of the knee and it feels relatively close to the skin surface.

Test

Stand about two feet away from a stool or a low chair. Put the foot of your injured leg on the stool or chair with your leg straight and your knee facing forward as shown. Relax your leg and place your hand on your outer thigh just above your knee. Press straight down (toward the floor) as hard as you can. Now repeat the test with your knee *slightly* bent (about one inch). Does either of these tests cause pain on the inner side of your knee?

If it does, you have verified a strain of this ligament. It should hurt you where you normally get your pain. If the injury is severe, you have to exert only a small amount of pressure, but if it's mild, don't be afraid to exert a lot of force.

Another test you can try is standing with your feet parallel and about twelve inches apart and drawing your knees together, which may also cause discomfort.

If no test hurts except pressing the inner knee with your finger, it may be a tiny bursa under the ligament that's at fault. This is a fairly rare problem, and requires treatment by injection.

This injury is often accompanied by a tear of the ligament that attaches your knee cartilage to the shinbone (the medial coronary ligament—see p. 125). These two lig-

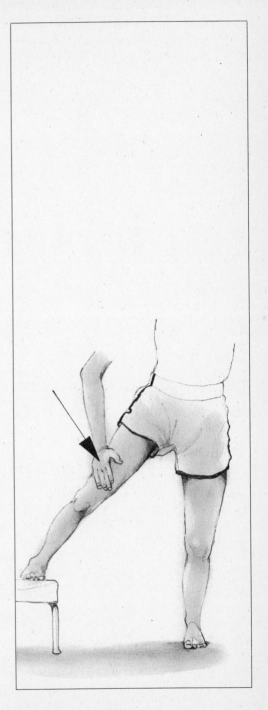

aments are often injured together because they are attached to each other. Also, if the knee is swollen, see p. 113.

TREATMENT CHOICES

Self-Treatment
If your knee swells a lot, it is a good idea to consult a physician to see if there's blood in the joint. Blood should always be removed immediately.

If you have a moderate strain with limited swelling, the swelling will go down slowly as the ligament heals. This might take a few months. In some cases there is no swelling at all. Rest the leg; do some ice treatment along with the Knee Extension exercise, p. 268, and bend and straighten your leg throughout the day as much as you can. This is to help prevent the scar tissue from adhering to the bone, where it shouldn't be.

I recommend getting some outside treatment on this injury because it can easily become chronic.

Medical Treatment
1. DEEP FRICTIONING: This is an effective treatment if done two or three times a week for three or four weeks. It speeds the healing of the ligament and prevents scar-tissue formation if done soon after the initial injury.

   In long-standing cases, treatment may take longer and should be combined with manipulation to free the ligament from the bone.
2. MANIPULATION: This is only effective where there is an adhesion. An inflamed ligament will not be helped by manipulation. It should be combined with other treatment when needed.
3. INJECTION: Corticosteroid injection is helpful in stopping inflammation and pain and preventing adhesions. It is also effective in the chronic stage when there are adhesions to the bone. The injection, when properly given, ruptures the adhesions and prevents additional adhesions from forming.

If the ligament has been excessively stretched and weakened, one or two injections of proliferant will help to tighten and strengthen it.

If the swelling is persistent beyond three months, a corticosteroid injection into the joint will eliminate the swelling in a few days.

4. CASTING: A plaster cast is often worn from the thigh to the ankle for three to six weeks, immobilizing the ligament so that it can heal. There are drawbacks to wearing the cast, however. The ligament may adhere to the bone beneath it, causing retears with strenuous physical activity. It can also result in a stiff knee.

5. SURGERY: If the ligament has been completely ruptured, surgical repair is best performed as soon as possible. After the initial recovery period, rehabilitative exercise therapy and deep massage should be started.

Rehabilitation
After your condition improves, try the first three Knee and Thigh exercises, pages 268–69.

Pain on the Outside of the Knee
(Lateral Collateral Ligament Tear)

WHAT IS IT?

Though this injury shares similarities with the medial, or inner, ligament tear (p. 116), it happens much less frequently and heals more easily. When this ligament (B in the drawing on page 122) is sprained or partially torn, some of its fibers separate and pain is distinctly felt on the outer side of the knee.

This ligament attaches the thigh bone to the outer-lower leg bone (C) (the fibula). It is less vulnerable to injury than its counterpart on the inner side of the knee because the

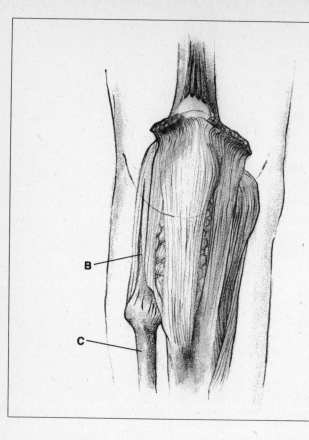

The lateral collateral ligament (B) attaches the thigh bone to the fibula (C)

knee is more stable on the outside. It helps guide the knee in a forward-backward direction and prevents it from buckling outward.

HOW AND WHY

This injury usually results from an accident, common in football, that involves a sudden blow to your inner knee. Or you could have a strange fall, where your knee buckles outward. If the knee is injured in this way it may swell and get warm and you may feel pain on the outer side. You can become prone to this injury by having overstretched ligaments on the outside of your knee. This frequently happens to people who practice yoga and spend a lot of time in the lotus position.

DIAGNOSTIC VERIFICATION

One of the clearest signs of this injury is the location of
pain on the outer side of the knee.

Test
Stand and rest the foot of your injured leg on the edge of a
chair. Your injured leg should be extended in front of you.
Turn your leg out as far as you can so the outer edge of
your foot is resting on the chair, as illustrated. Now place
both hands on the inner side of your knee and bend your
knee one to two inches. Press down toward the floor forcefully several times. If this ligament is injured there will be
pain on the outer side of the knee.

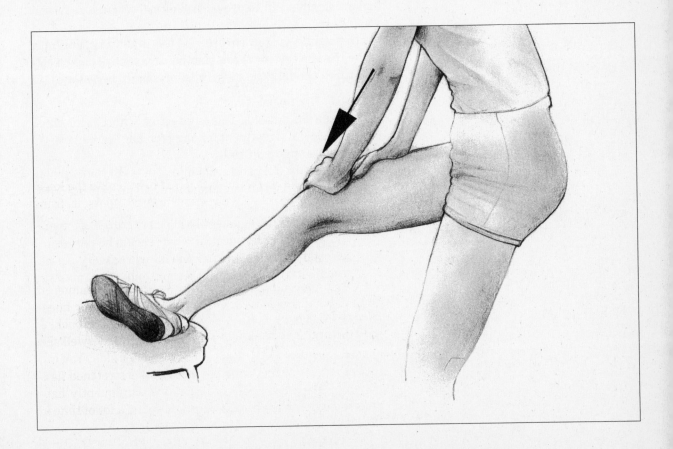

This injury may be confused with tensor fascia lata tendinitis (p. 94) and lateral coronary tear (p. 127). Try the tests for these injuries; if there is still some doubt about what your injury is, it may be that you have more than one. Consult a specialist if your pain doesn't get better in a few weeks.

TREATMENT CHOICES

Self-Treatment

Most self-treatment consists of waiting it out and limiting your activity, though ice treatment may help the injury heal more quickly. Bend and straighten your knee as fully as you can many times throughout the day to keep the ligament flexible and to prevent abnormal scar-tissue formation.

Depending on the severity of the injury, healing may take three weeks or three months. If you have completely ruptured the tendon, surgery is, of course, necessary.

Medical Treatment

1. DEEP FRICTIONING: This is effective with two or three weeks of treatment. Long-standing cases are, of course, more difficult.
2. INJECTION: Corticosteroid injection is very effective in stopping pain and inflammation and preventing adhesions.
3. SURGERY: If the ligament has been ruptured completely, which is rare, surgical repair should be performed as soon as possible. After the initial recovery period, rehabilitative exercise therapy and deep massage should be begun.

Rehabilitation

See the first four Knee and Thigh exercises, pages 268–69.

Pain on the Inner Side of the Knee, Slightly to the Front

(Medial Coronary Ligament Tear)

WHAT IS IT?

This is another extremely common knee injury, but it's often confused with a slightly torn cartilage (p. 106) or with a medial collateral ligament tear (p. 116). When this ligament (A) is injured, some of its fibers (B) have been strained and torn and the pain is felt slightly to the front of the inner side of the knee.

To find the location of this ligament, sit in a chair and bend your knee at a 90° angle. Place the tips of your middle and index fingers at the bottom of the kneecap, slightly toward the inside of the knee. With some pressure, move your fingers downward. You will feel a slight hollow and then hit a knob of bone that is like a shelf. On top of that bony shelf is where this ligament is found.

This ligament attaches the cartilage (meniscus) in your knee to the shinbone. Its function is to stabilize and control the movement of the thick, shock-absorbing cartilage (C) that lies within the knee.

Because this ligament is also attached to the medial collateral ligament (p. 116) they are often injured at the same time.

HOW AND WHY

This injury can be the result of accidents that force your leg to turn like a screwdriver—not one of its normal motions—which forces the knee to bend and twist inward. It can also occur from repeated running or jumping in poor alignment (knee turned inward, foot turned out); it happens as frequently in basketball and ballet as in football.

If you tear the cartilage in your knee, this ligament almost always tears as well. But more often, the ligament is torn and the cartilage is not, and this leads to understand-

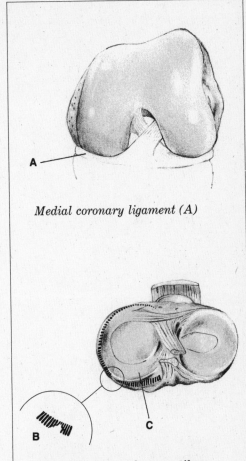

Medial coronary ligament (A)

The meniscus, or knee cartilage (C), and a tear (B) in the ligament that holds it in place

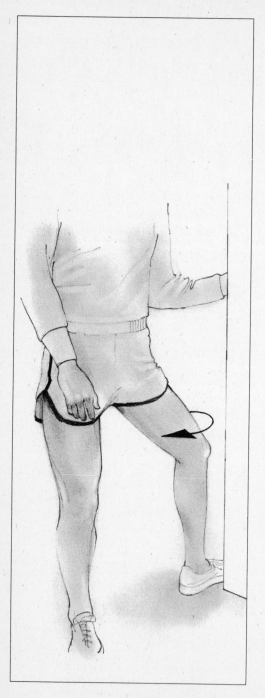

able confusion. To untangle the confusion, have the ligament treated first and wait and see.

If the injury occurs through an accident or fall, the pain is felt immediately and is horrendous. In severe sprains, swelling will occur within several hours, and it becomes difficult to walk for several days. In mild sprains there may not be swelling. As you're recovering you'll have pain any time you twist your knee or try to straighten your leg fully. With this injury you have the feeling that the leg is weak and going to give way, but this usually doesn't happen.

You can become vulnerable to this injury over time if you do the hurdler's stretch, fourth position on the floor in dance, or force your turnout in ballet. These things are not very good for the knee in general. If there is swelling, see p. 113.

DIAGNOSTIC VERIFICATION

A simple test for this injury is to do an old-time rock 'n' roll dance called the twist. This often causes pain in severe cases. A more definitive test uses more force.

Test
Stand facing an open door frame and place the inner arch of your foot flush against the doorjamb. Now bend your knee a few inches and turn your body away from the door frame as shown. The twisting motion that occurs in your knee should cause your pain. If that causes no discomfort, twist the knee forcefully and give it a slight jerk at the end.

This injury frequently accompanies a torn cartilage (p. 106), so be sure to check that section to understand the differences more fully.

TREATMENT CHOICES

Self-Treatment
With this ligament weakened, stress can easily be placed on the knee cartilage (the meniscus), so having it taken care of is important. Self-treatment is usually ineffective,

as rest is the only thing you can do, and this usually takes
two or three months. Maintain your strength by exercising while lying on the floor, so that the leg does not have to
bear weight. Be careful not to straighten the leg forcefully, for this will stress the ligament and prolong healing.
See a doctor.

Medical Treatment

1. DEEP FRICTIONING: This is successful with three or four
   weeks of intensive treatment, but only if strenuous
   activity is curtailed.
2. INJECTION: One or two injections of corticosteroid is
   usually effective in both recent and long-standing,
   chronic injuries. Only a small amount of medicine is
   needed, for this ligament is not very big.

   If at one time you had your meniscus removed and
   you still have a pain in the knee, your coronary ligament may have been torn as well and may not have
   healed. Injection is effective in this case also. Many
   patients suffer pain and disability for months and
   even years as a result of coronary ligament tears not
   dealt with after surgery. In some cases this leads to
   further surgery and/or the premature termination of
   an athletic or dance career.

   The use of proliferant injections where the ligament has been stretched and weakened strengthens
   and shortens the ligament, helps eliminate pain, and
   re-establishes the stability of the joint.

Rehabilitation

See Knee Extension and Up, Out, In, Down exercises,
pages 268, 269.

Outer Knee Pain, Slightly to the Front
(Lateral Coronary Ligament Tear)

WHAT IS IT?

No, a coronary ligament has nothing to do with a heart
attack! It's a skinny, flexible, wormlike ligament (A) on

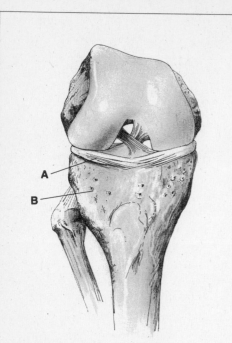

The coronary ligament (A) anchors the knee cartilage to the tibia (B)

the outer side of the knee. It holds the spongy, shock-absorbing, half-moon-shaped meniscus, or cartilage, in place, allowing it to slide forward and back while it serves as a cushion between the thigh bone and shinbone. This important ligament begins at the top of the shinbone (B) in the front of the knee and wraps around the knee toward the outside, anchoring the meniscus to bone (the tibia). When some of the ligament fibers are sprained and torn, pain can be sharp with sudden movement; however, the pain is usually of the dull-ache variety, either on the very outer side of the knee or slightly toward the front.

HOW AND WHY

Runners are very frequently afflicted with this injury along with football and basketball players. It's often an elusive, puzzling injury with many faces. In one instance, severe pain will come on only after three or four miles of running or forty-five minutes of a vigorous sport, disappearing a few hours later. In another case, pain will be constant and is intensified by just walking a few blocks. A sudden outward twist, with the foot and leg turning in, may cause a momentary buckling and feeling of weakness. This is followed by pain and/or swelling for several days or weeks. All of these symptoms point to the same common but often-missed injury: a lateral (outer) coronary ligament tear.

The danger of this injury is that it is often only one component of a more serious injury, a tear of the lateral meniscus (p. 106) usually referred to as a torn cartilage. When the cartilage is torn the knee periodically gives way, locks, and swells. While the ligament can be torn *without* the cartilage being damaged, an uncared-for injury to the ligament can lead to instability and a meniscal tear, which requires surgery.

How does it happen? It can occur slowly through the constant pounding of running on hard surfaces, particularly if you have poor knee/foot alignment (discussed on pp.

22–23). More frequently, it's dramatic and sudden. The foot is usually on the ground and there is a sudden forceful outward twist of the knee with the foot stationary (see diagnostic test drawing). The knee isn't designed to twist this way. What gives way first is the ligament, not the meniscus. I've seen this injury happen at basketball games where the player lands while turning in midair out of a jump shot. In football and soccer, too, this injury is easy to come by.

DIAGNOSTIC VERIFICATION

Test
Stand in an open doorway and place the outer side of the foot of the injured knee against the inner frame of the doorway, as illustrated. Now slowly twist the knee outward as far as you possibly can or until you feel your pain. The object of this test is to twist the knee outward without moving the foot. Use your hands and arms on the doorway to rotate and stabilize your body. Keep your injured leg relaxed—this means *you should not use the muscles in that leg.* In mild cases you need to give a little more force at the end of the twist to reproduce the pain. In extreme ones you only need to twist gently to feel the pain begin. Where a lot of exertion is needed before pain is felt, the tests may not work for you. In this case, see a professional. Also try your activity until you feel pain. Stop your activity and do the test immediately. If you don't feel the pain, it will be difficult for you or your doctor to find it conclusively with a positive test. Also see Torn Meniscus injuries, p. 106, and Water on the Knee, p. 113.

TREATMENT CHOICES

Self-Treatment
Ice treatment along with quadriceps exercises are often effective in mild and moderate injuries of this type. Limit your activities to those that produce no pain.

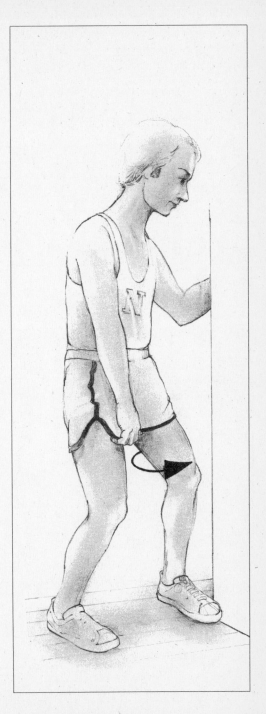

Rest! No dancing or sports except swimming.

Watch for involuntary leg collapsing and locking of the knee. If this happens, get to an orthopedist specializing in knees.

Medical Treatment

1. DEEP FRICTIONING: This method is effective when the tear is in the front portion of the ligament. When it's on the extreme outer side it cannot be reached by the finger. Treatment is a little painful and can take four or five weeks.

2. INJECTION: Corticosteroid injections are very effective with this injury. Proliferant injections are also effective. They strengthen the ligament when weakened. Proliferant is usually used a week or so after a steroid injection. If proliferant is used alone, healing time is longer.

Deep Knee Pain on Kneeling
(Bursitis of the Knee)

WHAT IS IT?

When people hear the word "bursitis" they imagine a shoulder that's stiff, painful, and hard to move. But bursas, those fluid-filled, crushable sacs, are all over the place, cushioning tendons and ligaments as they rub over bones. A very common place to have an irritated and swollen bursa (A) is in the knee. Pain can be intense or mild, depending on how inflamed the bursa is. The discomfort is usually felt as an ache, hard to pinpoint but most often perceived as originating deep inside the knee, below the kneecap.

There are several bursas located in the knee. The deep bursa (A) is very large and has three distinct sections: below the kneecap (1), under it (2), and above it (3). There is also a little bursa on top of the kneecap itself (B), and another one just below it (C), barely a quarter inch beneath

Right knee (side view) showing the deep bursa of the knee (A), the prepatellar bursa (B), and the superficial infrapatellar bursa (C)

the skin's surface. The common bursitis we will discuss here involves (1), the deep bursa below the kneecap.

HOW AND WHY

Anything I say on the causes of this injury is pure conjecture. I've never seen or heard of any research done on it. We do know, however, that if the bursa doesn't like something you did to it—a bad fall that brought you down on a bent knee, for example—it swells to protect itself against what you have done. When you kneel to pray or scrub it hurts; and squatting behind the batter's box is very painful also. In extreme cases, climbing stairs or walking can be an uncomfortable experience. The knee can sometimes appear swollen and feel a little hot, but it usually doesn't. Sometimes pain is felt right below the kneecap (C), just beneath the skin. Occasionally there is a swelling and tenderness right on top of the kneecap (B). And less frequently bursa (3) above the kneecap is painful and slightly hot. They all respond well to the treatment described at the end of this section.

Diagnosing bursas of the knee can be tricky. Sometimes patella tendinitis (strain of the tendon beneath the kneecap, p. 86) is present in addition to bursitis, confusing the issue for you. I remember seeing a thirty-five-year-old softball addict who hated injections. He had both of these injuries for eight months. It was only after many weeks of successful friction therapy on the tendon that it became clear his bursa was inflamed as well.

DIAGNOSTIC VERIFICATION

Test 1

Kneel on the bad knee only, allowing the knee to rest on the floor and keeping the thigh vertical; don't sit on your haunches. Do this on a hard floor, not a rug. Now, if it hasn't hurt yet, rock your weight slightly forward; this brings more weight directly onto the bursa. In moderate and severe cases this will hurt; in mild cases it may not.

Test 2

Now try a deep-knee bend on the balls of your feet. In most cases, when you reach the bottom of your knee bend there is pain.

Test 3

Now for the crucial test. Sit on the floor with your leg extended in front of you, as shown. Find your kneecap and place your thumb in the middle of the tendon that lies below it. (This is about half an inch below the kneecap toward the foot.) Be sure that your leg is fully relaxed. If the thigh muscles are contracted and the tendon is pulled tight the test will be ineffective. If you cannot straighten your knee, as is the case in a severe bursitis, do not try this test. (Also check Water on the Knee, p. 113).

Now if all is well so far, press your thumb down very forcefully toward the ground. In cases of bursitis, this is usually painful; you are pushing the tendon into the bursa, placing more stress on it, causing it to swell more and hurt.

TREATMENT CHOICES

Self-Treatment

This temperamental injury comes and goes as it pleases, getting worse and slightly better as if by whim. Rest, meaning eliminating or curbing activities that hurt, will occasionally help. But most often you are at the mercy of time. If untreated, this bursitis can last for years and years.

Medical Treatment

Manipulation does nothing for this injury and deep frictioning massage will usually make it worse.

The only treatment I know of that works is a corticosteroid injection. It usually takes only one to break the inflammation cycle, but three are sometimes needed. It works like a charm in three to five days. It is the most consistently successful injection in the knee.

The softball player I mentioned earlier had an injection

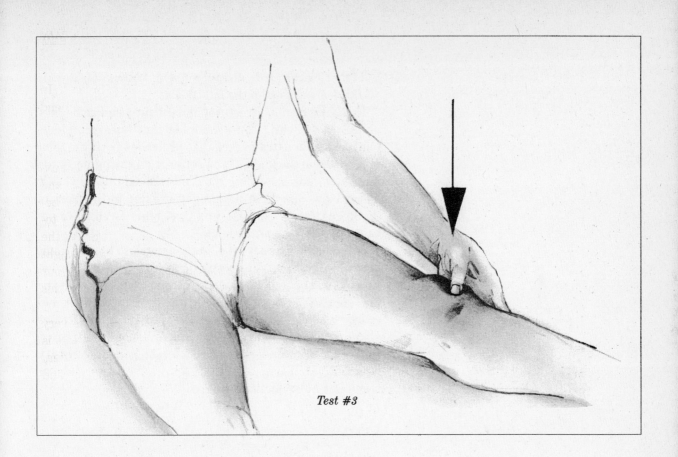

Test #3

after a little prodding and was happy and well in three days.

Swollen Back of the Knee
(Baker's Cyst)

"Look at that lump on the back of my knee," the patient anxiously says. "Yesterday I looked down and there it was. I'm terrified of lumps. My Aunt Mabel died of a lump."

The swelling the patient is concerned about is often the size of an egg. It's usually not painful and feels like a balloon filled with water. It causes a feeling of slight pressure and tautness behind the knee. This condition is called a

Baker's Cyst after its discoverer, Dr. William M. Baker, an English surgeon of the late 1800s.

It results from a structural abnormality that some people are born with. The membrane that lines your knee joint forms an extra pocket that protrudes from the joint at the back of the knee. If you suffer from any injury to the knee that causes swelling, fluid fills this additional pocket and it blows up. Most people get swelling in the front of the knee. People with Baker's Cyst often swell predominantly in the back of the knee.

A Baker's Cyst may be slightly annoying, but it's nothing to worry about. It doesn't do any good to drain it because it will only fill up again if you don't find and treat the precipitating injury that caused the swelling. This is because swelling is just a protective mechanism that comes along with many injuries. The *real* problem is a strain or tear of the cruciate ligament, collateral ligament, coronary ligament, cartilage, or the presence of a loose body or traumatic inflammation.

8

The Shoulder and Upper Arm

The tricky thing about evaluating your own shoulder injury is that it never hurts where it's supposed to. The other day I saw (for about the hundredth time) the confusion caused by referred shoulder pain. A young gymnast who was convinced that she had injured her biceps muscle just above the elbow came into the office of a physician friend of mine. She'd iced her biceps, stretched it, soaked it, and exercised it—all to no avail. She was surprised to learn that though her pain was in her biceps its cause was an injury to a tendon at the top of her shoulder about twelve inches away. Suddenly she understood why all her efforts had done no good.

Her story is not at all uncommon, for in all shoulder injuries except one the pain is felt not at the source of the injury but elsewhere. Usually the pain is felt in the upper arm, but at times it can be in the forearm and even (in some stranger cases) at the back of the shoulder. It's so hard to imagine this that people are usually skeptical and don't believe you until you've actually eliminated their pain.

135

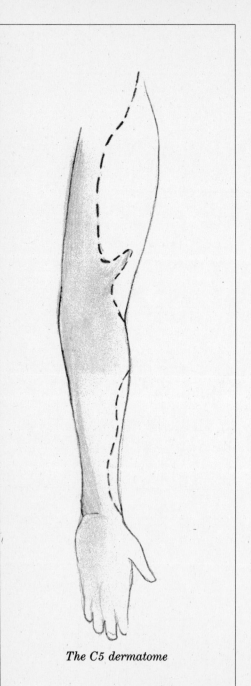

The C5 dermatome

To complicate this problem further, the five most common shoulder injuries all hurt in about the same place: in the middle of the upper arm. The more severe these injuries are, the farther they refer the pain toward the wrist.

In all injuries your brain helps you locate pain. With shoulder injuries your brain has a hard time. It should be feeling pain in the shoulder, but it's feeling it in the upper arm. This is because the structures of the shoulder (the shoulder joint, bursa, muscles, and most of the tendons) as well as the upper arm are developed from the same dermatome, called the C-5 dermatome.* It is as if these structures were fabricated from the same material and the brain cannot now differentiate between their different signals. Complicated and discouraging as it may sound, if you ignore where you feel the pain and focus on what actions cause the pain you can determine the source of your injury.

Remember that when you have a shoulder injury *some* movement of your arm is going to cause the pain; that is, unless you have upper-arm and shoulder pain that is actually caused by a neck injury. But all is not lost even in these cases. With a neck injury some movement of your head and neck, not your arm, will cause the pain in your shoulder or upper arm. If it's possible that you've injured your neck, do the tests for the neck, on p. 215, before testing your shoulder. Unfortunately, it is possible to have both a neck and shoulder injury at the same time. In this case you must seek professional help to untangle this mess.

The shoulder can move in more directions than any other joint in the body. Though this is a plus, it's also a minus because the greater the mobility, the greater the possibility of injury. Some of the shoulder's flexibility is due to its being a ball-and-socket mechanism and some to the way the arm is attached to the shoulder. Bones are usually held together by ligaments, but in the case of the shoulder this job is primarily done by muscles and tendons. Since the

*See pages 6–8.

tendons in the shoulder are doing not only their own job but the job of ligaments as well, they are easily strained and injured.

Several bones make up the shoulder. These include the upper arm bone, A in the illustration (the humerus); the collarbone, B (the clavicle); and the shoulder blade, C (the scapula), which contains the shoulder socket, D, a cuplike portion of the bone. The shoulder also has several joints. The joint most commonly referred to as the "shoulder joint" is the point at which the top of the arm fits into the shoulder socket. Most shoulder injuries occur where these two bones fit together.

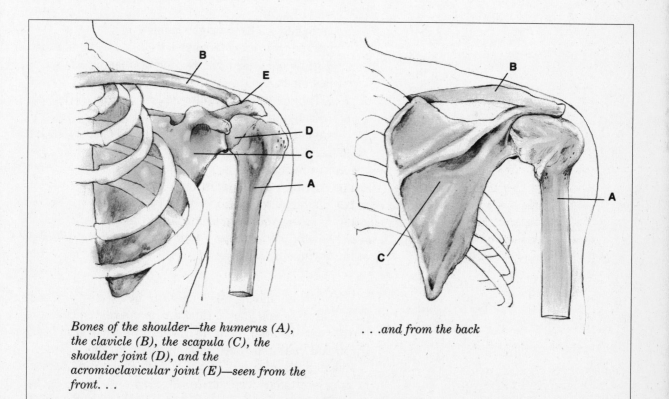

Bones of the shoulder—the humerus (A), the clavicle (B), the scapula (C), the shoulder joint (D), and the acromioclavicular joint (E)—seen from the front. . .

. . .and from the back

LOCATING YOUR INJURY

There is no way around it, finding and identifying your shoulder injuries will be a bit tougher than finding other injuries because of the referred pain. I can't give you diagrams to indicate what injury is where, but since particular movements can aid in identifying your injury the following list may help. If any of these movements are painful or cause you difficulty, turn to the appropriate page:

1. Forehand in tennis or tennis serve   p. 144
2. Backhand in tennis   150
3. Dumbbell curl   153
4. Reaching from the front seat to the back
   seat of a car   150
5. Imbedding a screw right-handed or
   removing a screw left-handed   153
6. Tightening a jar right-handed or opening a
   jar left-handed   153
7. Lifting or holding a suitcase   147
8. Lifting your arm above
   shoulder height   139, 156, 160, 163
9. Lying on your bad shoulder   156, 160
10. Throwing a ball   144
11. Putting a coat or shirt on   150
12. Pulling a sweater over your head   150
13. If lifting your arm is impossible and there is
    severe pain or a deep ache in the shoulder 156, 160
14. Swimming the crawl   144

With one shoulder injury there is never any referred pain. This is a pain you'd feel at a very specific point at the top of your shoulder, E, p. 137, where your ear would rest if you laid your head onto your shoulder, p. 139.

Rehabilitation exercises are a very important part of getting over shoulder injuries. Be sure to read the entire Rehabilitation chapter so you know how to use the exercises given later.

Point of the Shoulder Pain

(Acromioclavicular Joint)

WHAT IS IT?

Let's start with the easiest first, the injury with no referred pain. This injury can be readily found because the
pain is where it should be, at point A, and the trouble
stems from a tiny joint at the top of the shoulder. There
are two causes for pain at this point, a sprain of the ligament holding these two bones together (B) or an irritation
inside the joint, which lies under the ligament.

This joint is formed by the joining of the collar bone and

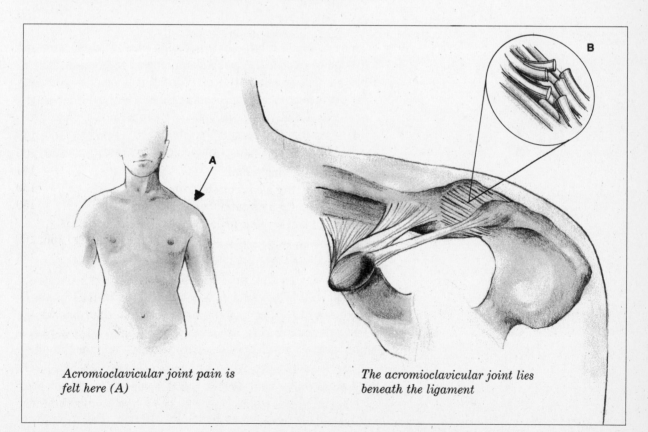

Acromioclavicular joint pain is
felt here (A)

The acromioclavicular joint lies
beneath the ligament

the upper part of the shoulder blade (see illustrations on page 137). Most people think of their shoulder blades as being in their backs, but parts of it go to the front of the body as well. The scapula bone is one of the strangest looking bones there is. To find this joint, place your fingers on your collar bone and follow it out toward the tip of your shoulder. Where your collar bone ends there's a tiny little groove. This is where the joint is.

Football fans know their man is in big trouble if the announcer says he's suffered a shoulder separation. In this severest form of the injury, always caused by some accident, the joint is torn apart, leaving a gap between the two bones. When this happens you suffer enormous pain all over the shoulder.

HOW AND WHY

This is a small, relatively weak joint which is vulnerable as it is quite exposed. A very common way to injure it is in a bicycle fall, or as a result of a direct blow or fall—you can hurt it in a car accident, or in a collision with another player in basketball. But it can also happen with strenuous lifting or with push-ups and chin-ups.

This injury can hang around forever, getting better or worse with the degree of activity performed.

DIAGNOSTIC VERIFICATION

If you've had a severe accident and think you may have injured your point-of-the-shoulder joint, it is important to get an X ray. It's important that this X ray is done in a special way that shows if the bones have been separated. You should be given a five-pound weight to hold in your hand, and the X ray should be taken from the front while you're standing. The use of the weight makes the separation clearer. Both shoulders are usually done for the purpose of comparison when the separation is very small. If the shoulder is separated, there is usually a gap at the very end of the collar bone and it is almost impossible to lift your arm over your head. In addition, Test 1, shown below, is very painful and almost impossible to do all the way.

Test 1
Place the arm of the injured shoulder straight out in front of you. Put the palm of the other hand around your elbow, as shown. Now, using your good arm, draw the extended arm toward your opposite shoulder. Do this slowly, with a fair amount of force. If you have this injury, this movement usually causes more pain than the movements given in the tests that follow. In most people, at least two out of the following three tests also cause pain.

Test 2
Place your injured arm straight above your head. Take the hand of the other arm and place it on your elbow. With the

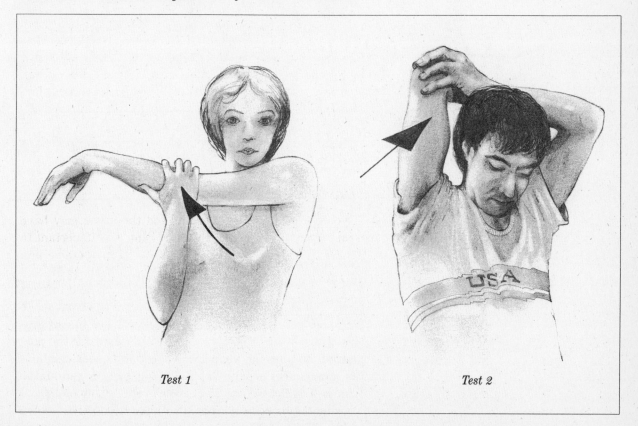

Test 1   *Test 2*

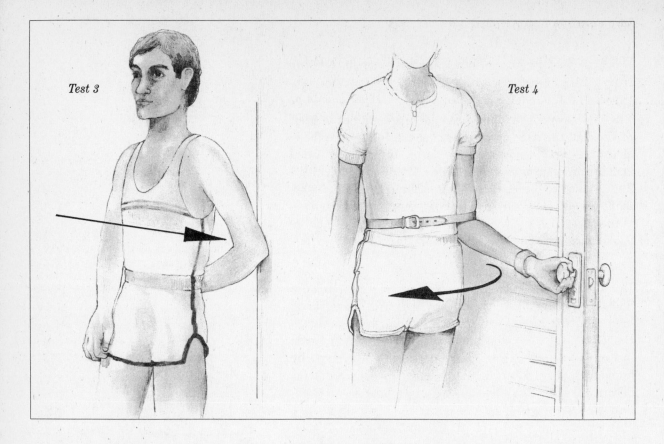

Test 3

Test 4

good hand holding the weight of your arm, push the arm backward as far as it will go, three or four times. Does that cause you pain?

Test 3
Place the hand of your injured shoulder behind your back so that the back of your wrist is resting against the upper part of the buttock. Stand in an open doorway, place the inside of your elbow against the side doorjamb, and lean back so that your arm rotates inward. Be sure to relax your arm. Sometimes this one doesn't hurt.

Test 4
Place a belt around your lower chest and arm so as to fix the upper arm of your injured shoulder into your body. The belt should come just above your elbow. Facing a doorknob, grasp the doorknob with the hand of the injured

shoulder. Letting your arm relax, rotate your body *away* from the door, so that the arm of your injured shoulder approaches a 180° angle with your body. The belt should be tight enough to keep your upper arm at the side of your body. Stretch as far as you can and see if that causes you some discomfort.

In the previous three tests the discomfort is felt at the very end of the test movement. If the result was vague, give the arm an extra stretch at the end of the test.

TREATMENT CHOICES

Self-Treatment

In minor strains, resting the arm for three to six weeks will sometimes effect a cure, but more often the pain will linger on. Ice treatment is effective in some cases. With the ice use the Forehand Lift, exercise B. There are even instances when shoulder separations have been fixed by immediate ice treatment accompanied by movement (as described on pp. 31–32) done for many hours a day for several weeks.

It is best to see a physician if your pain doesn't disappear quickly (say in three or four weeks). Massage and manipulation do nothing for it. If your pain is severe, get to a doctor right away.

Medical Treatment

1. INJECTION: In both joint inflammation and ligament strain, corticosteroid injections are the most effective treatment. Injections are effective within a few days. Within two weeks you should be able to resume full activity.

    Proliferant injections are very helpful when there is a shoulder separation. They help the new tissue to form more quickly in the healing process and render you pain free in a fraction of the time that other treatments take.
2. SURGERY: If the joint is torn completely loose, surgery is usually necessary.

Rehabilitation

If you have had this injury for a while, many shoulder muscles will weaken. Try all of the Shoulder and Upper-Arm exercises (pp. 270–72) when you begin to feel better.

Tennis Serve and Forehand Pain
(Subscapularis Tendinitis)

WHAT IS IT?

It's amazing how common this injury is and how frequently it's misunderstood. If your shoulder has been hurt there's a 70 to 85 percent chance that this is what you've got. When your subscapularis tendon (A) is injured, some of its fibers are strained and torn. Pain is felt in the upper arm but can be referred down as far as the wrist if the strain is severe. When the tear is in the muscle (B), which is rare, pain is felt underneath the shoulder blade.

The subscapularis muscle is very strong. It is attached to the under-surface of the shoulder blade, sandwiched between the shoulder blade and the ribs. Its tendon attaches to the top of the arm on the inside (C). It's hard to visualize because the tendon goes through your body from back to front. This is the muscle that helps you open jars, swim the crawl, lift things, throw a ball, and complete the forehand and serving actions in tennis and other racquet sports.

HOW AND WHY

This injury almost always makes its appearance slowly. Gradually you find that lifting your hand above your head hurts; or after about a half hour of playing tennis, serving brings on a general ache in your shoulder and possibly a pain down the back of your upper arm. If it's really bad, opening a jar with the right hand will be painful, as will opening a door. Throwing a ball around for a while can also bring on this pain, as this is the main muscle used in pitching, both overhand and side-arm. That is why so many

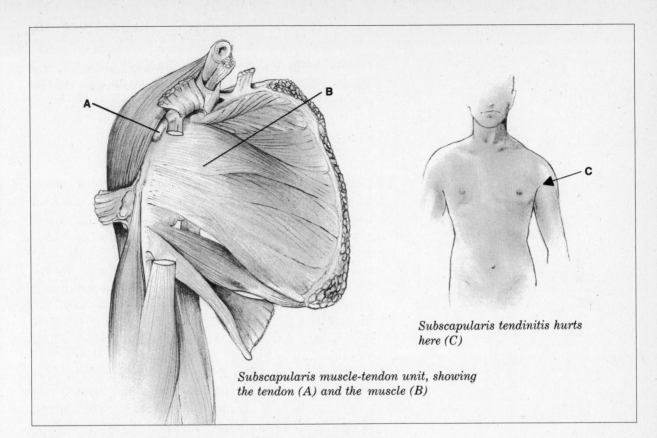

Subscapularis tendinitis hurts
here (C)

Subscapularis muscle-tendon unit, showing
the tendon (A) and the muscle (B)

pitchers suffer from this injury. I've seen many people
over the years who've resigned themselves to pain during
the softball season, when a little bit of treatment and self-
care would clear it up. It's hard to know the exact cause,
for the pain is often felt several days after the strain has
occurred.

Poor or insufficient warm-up exercises before racquet
sports or throwing sports is a common cause of this injury—with a good warm-up, the muscle-tendon unit is more
pliable and can absorb stress more easily. Overdoing it,
especially after a lay-off, will also make you vulnerable.

This injury tends to become chronic, coming and going
with the amount of exertion you perform. Each new exertion creates a small tear that heals with adherent scar tissue. The scar tissue tears *again* with each new stressful
activity. This cycle can occur a hundred times in a few
months, creating a matted scar which is painful and weak.

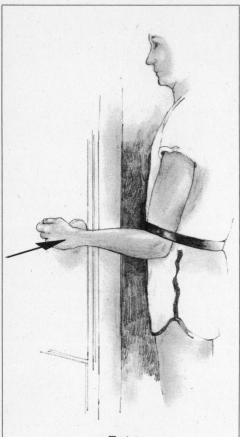

Test 1

Over a period of time, the muscle works inefficiently and becomes weakened, although you may not notice this because of the tremendous strength of this muscle.

DIAGNOSTIC VERIFICATION

Test 1
To test for subscapularis tendinitis efficiently, you need to fix your upper arm to your body. Tie a belt around your lower chest so that the upper arm (just above the elbow) of your injured shoulder is held firmly to your body, as illustrated. Stand in an open doorway facing the doorjamb and place a ball between the wrist of your injured arm and the doorjamb. Your arm should be held in front of you and you should be facing the ball. Now press your wrist into the ball with all of your might, as if hitting a forehand on the tennis court. If that did not cause discomfort, rotate your body away from the ball a quarter of a turn so that your lower arm is held out to your side. From this position push your wrist into the ball forcefully. That should create pain somewhere in the upper arm if you have this injury. If your injury is very slight, the next test may be the only one that will make it clear.

Test 2
Staying in the position just described, with your upper arm to the side, release pressure on the ball, rest the wrist, relax your arm muscles, and rotate your body even further than the 90°, forcing your shoulder muscles to stretch. In mild cases this should produce pain. If pain is felt in the upper arm during this or the previous test, the tendon is probably injured where it attaches to the upper-arm bone. If pain is felt under the shoulder blade as you perform the test, the muscle has been injured.

TREATMENT CHOICES

Self-Treatment
If the strain is mild, a week or two of rest, along with ice treatment and the Forehand Lift exercises as described on

pp. 270–71, may be curative. Unfortunately, most of these injuries undergo repeated tearing and poor scar-tissue formation and need medical treatment.

Medical Treatment
1. DEEP FRICTIONING: This somewhat painful but effective treatment usually takes three to four weeks.
2. INJECTION: One or two corticosteroid injections are usually effective within a week or two, but they should be followed by several weeks of rehabilitative exercise. Proliferant injections are also effective, but the healing time is four to six weeks.

Rehabilitation
Do the Forehand Lift A and B with light weights, pp. 270–71.

Pain When Lifting a Suitcase
(Supraspinatus Tendinitis)

WHAT IS IT?

Walking around Europe with a heavy suitcase is one of the more enjoyable ways to get this injury. When it's really bad, discomfort can be referred all the way down to the hand. In milder cases the pain stays in the upper arm. Athletes and older individuals can suffer severe injury: the tendon is sometimes completely ruptured and it is impossible to lift your arm from your side. (If this occurs, see a surgeon immediately.)

This small muscle runs along the upper portion of the shoulder blade (A) and attaches to the top of the arm (B). This is where the tendon fibers that are usually strained tear; the tendon also tears where it attaches to the muscle (C). The muscle allows you to move your arm away from the side of your body up to about twelve inches before other muscles take over that action. You use it especially when carrying a suitcase, trying to prevent it from banging into the outside of your knee.

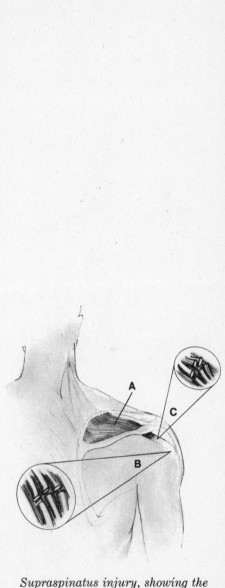

Supraspinatus injury, showing the muscle (A), the tendon attachment (B), and the muscle-tendon juncture (C)

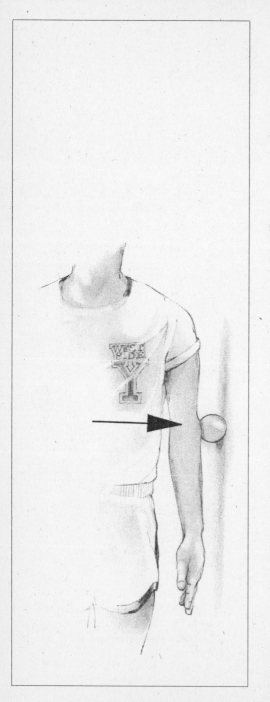

HOW AND WHY

This injury usually occurs out of the blue—it's hard to say what causes it exactly, except that the muscle (A) is weak in most people and it is sometimes called on to do sudden, very strenuous activity it is unaccustomed to doing. You can hurt yourself as easily scrubbing a pot with unusual vigor or mopping a floor as you can in athletic activity.

Or you might be injured by a severe fall, where the hand is placed in front of you to break the fall. Whatever the case, the pain is usually felt several hours after strenuous activity, as with many tendon strains, and you may experience it when the arm is extended at shoulder height out from the side of the body, or when reaching high over your head. This injury can persist for ten years if not treated.

DIAGNOSTIC VERIFICATION

Test

To test for this injury you need a ball or something round that will offer you some resistance. With your ball, or whatever, in hand, stand sideways about three inches away from a wall with your injured shoulder nearest the wall. With your feet about a foot apart, place the ball between the wall and your elbow (your elbow should now be out about two or three inches from your body). Now, without moving the rest of your body, press your upper arm into the ball as hard as you can. If it causes you discomfort *while you are pushing*, you have injured the supraspinatus tendon. But if it causes pain *after* you release your pressure, you most probably have a subscapularis tendon tear (see p. 144) or an infraspinatus tendon injury (see p. 150). If you cannot push out at all, you have ruptured the tendon completely.

If a serious fall or trauma brought on your injury, it is wise to have an X ray to see if you have fractured any bones. When the X ray is read, deposits of calcium are sometimes found in the supraspinatus tendon. It is often assumed that these deposits, rather than an inflammation in the tendon, are the cause of pain, and surgery is at times recommended. Supraspinatus pain that is due to calcium deposits is rare. There are simply calcium deposits present in addition to the tendon strain.

TREATMENT CHOICES

Self-Treatment

If your strain is minor, several weeks' rest will probably take care of it; but if it is severe or if poor scar-tissue formation has occurred, your discomfort may go on indefinitely. If you're not better within two to four weeks, seek medical treatment.

Medical Treatment

The supraspinatus can be torn in three separate places. In order for medical treatment to be effective, the physician or therapist will have to locate the exact place of the tear.

1. DEEP FRICTIONING: I have personally used this method with great success. Although it is somewhat painful, it is very effective within several weeks.
2. INJECTION: Corticosteroid injection is also quite effective with this injury, although it sometimes takes several injections to complete the job. A good friend of mine had supraspinatus pain for five years. When nothing anyone could do seemed to help him, I suggested he get injections. To his surprise, the injections gave him almost 100 percent relief. He had had injections many years before by his family doctor, who had not understood the referred-pain phenomenon. Injecting the arm where he felt the pain could do no good, of course, because the tear was four inches higher. If your physician is not sure which spot is injured, have him perform a test injection with a local anaesthetic. Two minutes after the injection, take out your ball and retest your arm. If the pain is gone, he's got the right spot. If it isn't, you'll have to try again.
3. SURGERY: When the supraspinatus tendon is completely torn and you cannot lift your arm away from

your side at all, surgical repair is the only thing that will restore it to its natural function. In order for this operation to be successful, it needs to be done as soon after the injury as possible, preferably within days. This is usually a successful operation, especially in younger people.

Rehabilitation
See Weighted Arm Circle, p. 272.

Backhand Pain
(Infraspinatus Tendinitis)

WHAT IS IT?

I got this injury after slamming a baseball over a roof, and it stayed with me a year, defying all attempts at diagnosis and treatment. This injury interfered with lots of activities—even my sleep. I couldn't put my shirt on without pain.

The infraspinatus muscle-tendon unit is used in a backhand motion, when writing, and when reaching behind you. The muscle covers the lower portion of the shoulder blade, and its tendon attaches to the very top of your arm in the back (A). When you have infraspinatus tendinitis, pain is felt in the upper-arm region, sometimes slightly to the back. If your injury is severe, the pain is referred down the top of the arm to the wrist, but this occurs only in extreme cases.

HOW AND WHY

This tendon strain often occurs in racquet sports and tends to come on slowly. Some people even have a minor strain of the tendon which continues unnoticed for years. There might be a slight discomfort when reaching for something on a high shelf or in the back seat of your car—but this discomfort can set the stage for a more severe injury later on.

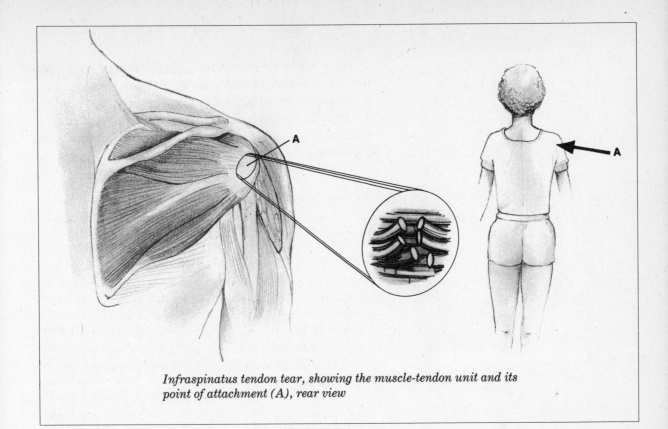

Infraspinatus tendon tear, showing the muscle-tendon unit and its point of attachment (A), rear view

When a severe strain of the tendon occurs, you frequently feel nothing because the tendon is warmed up; later that day or the next morning you may have difficulty putting on your shirt or your coat, as you lift your arm up and to the side. This muscle is pretty weak in most people. So, if called on to perform heavy exertion suddenly, it can easily strain and tear. It can be a very nasty and tenacious injury.

DIAGNOSTIC VERIFICATION

Test 1
To verify this injury we have to isolate the infraspinatus. You'll need a ball and a belt. First, place the belt around your lower chest, tying your injured arm to your body just above the elbow. Make sure to buckle it tight enough to

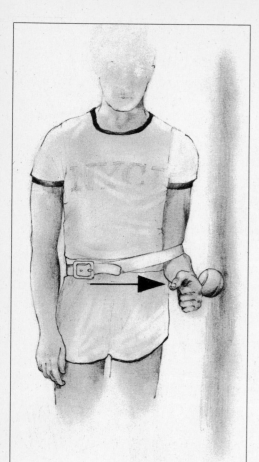

Test 1

prevent your elbow from moving away from your side. Now stand sideways with your injured arm next to a wall. With your elbow at a right angle, place the ball between the wall and the back of your wrist. Push the ball into the wall with the back of your wrist with all the strength you can muster.

Test 2
If Test 1 does not re-create your discomfort, turn your body toward the wall so that your hand is about six inches from your belly and try it again.

Test 3
Rotate your body away from the wall, beyond your original sideways position, as if you were near the end of a backhand swing, and push from this position.

Don't forget, the belt is a very important part of the test, and without it misdiagnosis is almost guaranteed. If you have infraspinatus tendinitis, one of these tests should cause you pain.

TREATMENT CHOICES

Self-Treatment
Hitting backhand is out, as well as any exercise that gives you pain. I would especially stay away from push-ups and chin-ups. Two to three months of rest sometimes will allow the injury to heal, but more often it will stay around for years, especially if you are active. Do the ice treatment along with the Backhand Lift if you can do so without pain. Medical treatment is usually recommended if rest and ice don't work.

Medical Treatment
1. DEEP FRICTIONING: Several weeks of treatment usually are effective if the tendon tear is not too widespread. Three to four weeks are generally required.
2. INJECTION: One or two corticosteroid injections are usually effective. This should be followed by several days' rest and a week or two of rehabilitation.

One or two injections of proliferant are effective in chronic cases or where cortisone has failed. The proliferant stimulates the build-up of strength in the tendon, so six to eight weeks may be required for a good result. The rehabilitation exercises outlined should be used during this period.

Rehabilitation
See the Backhand Lift and the Weighted Arm Circle exercises, pp. 271–72.

Chin-Up Pain
(Biceps Tendinitis)

WHAT IS IT?

Kids are always asking each other to "make a muscle"; then they carefully compare the size and hardness of their biceps. The bigger the better. This is the muscle that helps you bend your elbow and rotate your forearm outward—as when closing a jar with your right hand. When you injure your biceps, some of the fibers of this complex muscle-tendon unit have been torn, and there is pain in the upper arm with certain movements. The biceps muscle actually has two parts, which are attached to a common tendon that starts just below the elbow on your forearm (B). What makes the biceps muscle complex is that it splits into two separate muscles as it travels up toward the shoulder. The short part (A) has its own tendon, which attaches just above the armpit. The tendon of the longer part of the muscle (C) does a totally unique dive through your shoulder joint and attaches toward the back of it deep beneath the surface. The biceps muscle crosses over two different joints, the elbow and the shoulder, whereas most muscles cross only one. This double-crossing means that your pain could either be in your upper arm, near the shoulder or down near your elbow, depending on where you've injured this muscle-tendon unit.

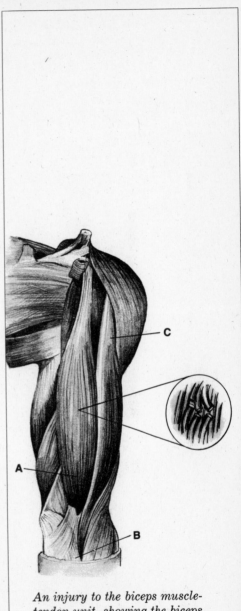

An injury to the biceps muscle-tendon unit, showing the biceps short head (A), the lower tendon (B), and the biceps long head (C)

The biceps can be injured in several places when there is pain in the upper arm. The belly of the muscle can be strained, but this is rare. Most frequently, it's the tendon, just above where the muscle ends or in a part of the tendon that goes through the shoulder joint.

HOW AND WHY

People who enjoy lifting weights, or who frequently have to lift heavy objects as part of their work, are quite susceptible to this injury. It's also common in people who have decided to be their own mover, not realizing how heavy their furniture is. If you are right-handed, you might notice that closing jars tightly, or using a screwdriver to tighten a screw, causes pain. (If you're left-handed, opening jars and unscrewing screws will cause the pain.) This injury is less common than others we've been talking about, and it usually happens if you push further when fatigued, or when you drop something heavy—such as your end of the piano—and need to catch it quickly.

DIAGNOSTIC VERIFICATION

Test 1
Stand next to a door and grip the doorknob with your palm directly under the knob. While holding the doorknob, without gripping too tightly, try to lift your hand toward the ceiling with a great deal of force. Does that cause you pain? If it does, you need to do one more test to confirm that it's your biceps and not another muscle that's injured.

Test 2
Hold your injured arm in front of your chest with your elbow bent, palm facing the floor. Grip your wrist strongly with the other hand. Resisting the movement firmly with the hand of your good arm, try to rotate your forearm outward forcefully. If your biceps is injured, this will cause pain.

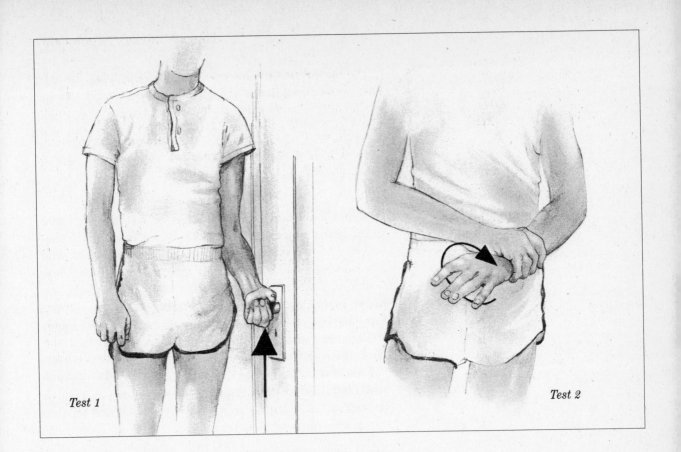

Test 1   Test 2

TREATMENT CHOICES

Self-Treatment
Rest, along with ice therapy and the Biceps Curl (p. 272),
will often get you over a minor strain, but some tendon
strains can be quite long-lasting if not medically treated.

Medical Treatment
1. DEEP FRICTIONING AND DEEP MASSAGE: These treatments
   are effective when the tear has occurred in the muscle or the part of the tendon that is easily accessible.
   They don't work if it's in the part of the tendon that
   penetrates the shoulder joint.
2. INJECTION: Corticosteroid injections are effective
   when any part of the biceps is injured and inflamed

but difficult to inject precisely in the tendon where it goes through the shoulder joint.

Rehabilitation
See Biceps Curl (p. 272). Also try holding a five- or eight-pound weight and slowly rotating your forearm inward and outward.

Severe Shoulder Pain
(Acute Bursitis)

WHAT IS IT?

If you see stars from the pain of lifting your arm you may well have acute bursitis, the most painful shoulder injury. There are two kinds of bursitis, acute and chronic. I have put them in two separate sections because everything about them is different. In acute bursitis there is severe swelling and inflammation of the bursa sac within the shoulder, and extreme pain in the upper arm and shoulder area. Sometimes this pain extends all the way down the arm.

The bursa within the shoulder joint is a fluid-filled sac, like a plastic bag half filled with water, which cushions the tendons as they slide over rough-surfaced bones. It's about the size of a tangerine, and it adapts its shape in response to the movements you make with your arm.

HOW AND WHY

This injury sneaks up on you over a few days. In the beginning there is usually a dull pain that appears in the shoulder or upper arm for no apparent reason. Over the next day or two the pain becomes more intense and constant and may travel down your arm. Moving the arm is agony for a couple of weeks, and it is practically impossible to lie on that shoulder. If you do nothing but wait, the pain begins to diminish after a few weeks. After three or four

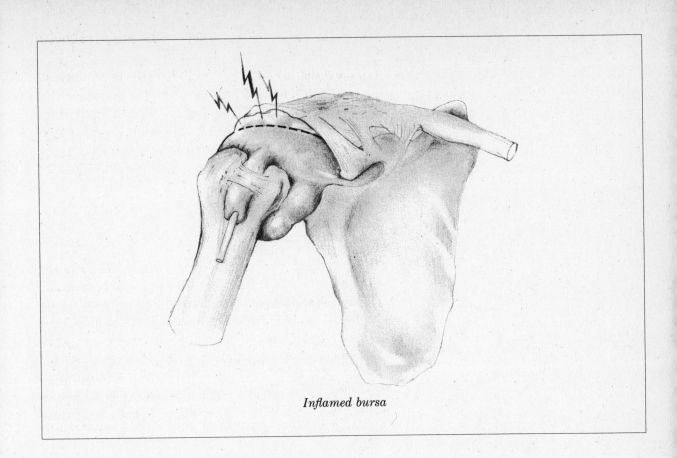

Inflamed bursa

weeks, you can lift your arm with only slight pain, and by the end of six to eight weeks it's usually gone.

No one knows what causes bursitis, but it is likely that some slight trauma irritates the bursa and the only thing it knows how to do to protect itself is swell so badly that any movement compresses it, causing excruciating pain. But this is just speculation. This sort of bursitis tends to recur every few years in some individuals.

DIAGNOSTIC VERIFICATION

There are no diagnostic tests for acute bursitis that you can easily do yourself. The way the pain progresses and the intensity of it are your best clues. Acute bursitis is often confused with several different arthritic conditions, especially the one described on p. 160. The only way to tell the difference yourself is to compare the histories carefully and see if you can puzzle it out. Isolating the differences with testing procedures is a subtle business, but a physician can readily do it. The main difficulty is lifting your arm out to the side.

TREATMENT CHOICES

Self-Treatment
The only thing you can do yourself is rest. Massage and manipulation will irritate bursitis. Ice may temporarily make you feel more comfortable but doesn't speed the recovery.

Medical Treatment
Painkilling drugs can minimize the pain you feel during the course of healing. Corticosteroid injections given along with a local anaesthetic will get rid of the inflammation within two to three days. Be prepared to feel a little worse the next day from the injection.

Pain in the Back of the Upper Arm
(Triceps Injury)

WHAT IS IT?

This is a horrible injury for those who like to elbow their way through crowds. Rush-hour subway riders who have it have to find another way to get a seat, and devoted stick-shift drivers suddenly wish they had an automatic. With this injury you will feel pain in the back of the upper arm if you have injured the muscle fibers (A). If the tendon (B) of your triceps muscle is injured, your pain will be in the back of the arm just above the elbow. This muscle-tendon unit begins behind the elbow and has a wide flat tendon. As it travels up toward the back of the shoulder it

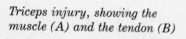

Triceps injury, showing the muscle (A) and the tendon (B)

splits into three separate muscles, each with its own tendon that attaches behind the shoulder. Fortunately, the upper tendons rarely get injured, for when they do they are more difficult to locate and treat.

HOW AND WHY

Khrushchev used this muscle when he was pounding his shoe at the U.N. More conventional uses include hammering, pulling back on your stick shift, and jabbing people with your elbow. You usually injure it only when you really overdo it playing softball, chopping wood, or lifting heavy weights above your head. It can also come out of the blue. A friend of mine injured her triceps while shifting gears with no extra stress involved. This injury rarely refers pain; it hurts where you are injured and usually only when you're actually using that muscle. If you injure the muscle itself you tend to heal rather quickly. Injuries to the tendon near the elbow are much more stubborn.

DIAGNOSTIC VERIFICATION

Test
Stand sideways with your injured arm next to a closed door. Now grip the doorknob from the top so that your palm faces the floor. Try to push the doorknob down to the floor. Exert as much force as you can. Does that cause you any discomfort? If it does you've injured your triceps muscle or tendon.

TREATMENT CHOICES

Self-Treatment
Ice treatment to the painful part of the back of the arm— along with Triceps Extension exercise—are often effective. This injury should clear up in about a week or two.

Medical Treatment
1. DEEP FRICTIONING AND DEEP MASSAGE: Both of these are very effective treatments.

2. INJECTION: If you have a stubborn case where the lower tendon is injured, corticosteroid or proliferant injections are very effective treatments.

Rehabilitation
See Triceps Extension exercise, p. 272.

Stiff Painful Shoulder
(Traumatic Arthritis of the Shoulder)*

WHAT IS IT?

For some unknown reason if you're a woman in your forties you are tremendously prone to this injury. You don't have to do anything more extraordinary than bumping into a wall to get this one. At first you feel a dull, aching pain around your shoulder and/or in your arm. This pain gets progressively more intense. What's happened is that your shoulder joint has become inflamed.

The shoulder is a ball-and-socket joint and is supposed to move in more directions than any other joint in the body. The joint is surrounded by thousands of tough fibers (A) that contain a lubricating fluid which permits ease in movement. When the shoulder has been traumatized in some way many of the shoulder-joint fibers within the joint (B) shrink, making any movement that stretches them extremely painful.

HOW AND WHY

Traumatic arthritis is unusual because it has a very definite pain cycle. It runs a course from nine to twelve months in three segments that can last three to four

---

*Arthritis means a shrinking of the joint capsule. There are many kinds of arthritis. The one induced by a trauma is the least serious and easiest to treat.

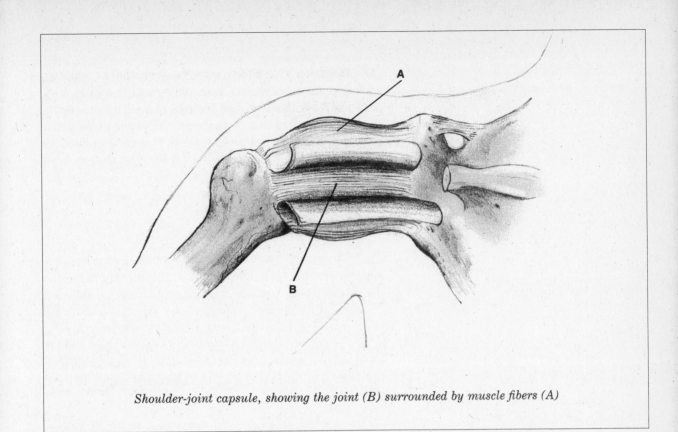

Shoulder-joint capsule, showing the joint (B) surrounded by muscle fibers (A)

months. To begin it, you usually bump into something and you might not even notice it. Generally it hurts a bit for a day and then disappears, only to return about three or four days later. During the first three-month cycle the pain continues to increase and your ability to move your arm decreases. Reaching around to wash your back or to zip up a dress, brushing your hair or lifting your arm over-head gradually becomes impossible. In addition to less-ened mobility, you experience the following three things: first, it's extremely painful to lie on the injured shoulder at night; second, the shoulder begins to hurt continually even without movement; and last, a referred pain slowly travels down the arm and can even reach the wrist.

During the second three- or four-month period the pain gradually lessens and retreats back up to the shoulder. It's easier to lie on your bad side and your shoulder hurts only with specific movements. Your movement is still limited, particularly in moving your arm above your head or out to the side. The muscles have their own check-and-balance system and will suddenly contract to prevent you from doing something that could further injure your shoulder.

During the last three- or four-month phase full movement usually returns and the arm gets better by itself.

DIAGNOSTIC VERIFICATION

There are many types of arthritis, so have a physician examine your shoulder. The onset and the ensuing pattern is the primary way you'll be able to evaluate your shoulder. One symptom definitely occurs: you absolutely can't lift your arm straight up above your head. The testing for this injury is unfortunately too difficult to do on your own. In addition, traumatic arthritis is frequently confused with the two types of bursitis of the shoulder, pages 156 and 163. So see a doctor.

TREATMENT CHOICES

Self-Treatment
This is a case where time alone will heal your ills if you are the patient type who can stand to wait out the nine to twelve months that it takes.

Medical Treatment
1. STRETCHING THE SHOULDER: This technique must be performed by a physical therapist and is an effective treatment only if you begin it within a few weeks of the time the injury begins. It also works in the last three- or four-month phase of the injury. The timing is important because in the beginning and ending phases your body is more receptive to this treatment. Three weeks of stretching will stop the cycle in either phase.
2. INJECTION AND STRETCHING: Injections of corticoste-

roids will halt the pain cycle at any point. The injections are most effective when combined with
Stretching the shoulder, described above. You can
do the stretching at any phase of the injury as long as
it's coupled with the injections. You may need two or
three injections to do the job.

Rehabilitation

All the muscles weaken with this injury. Try all of the
Shoulder and Upper Arm exercises, pp. 270–72, for several months.

NOTE: Deep massage, frictioning, and manipulation *are
not helpful with this problem*. In fact, manipulation might
make it much worse.

Mild Shoulder Ache When Lifting the Arm
(Chronic Bursitis)

WHAT IS IT?

If you are worried that the mild and erratic ache in your
shoulder is arthritis, you may be happy to learn you might
have chronic bursitis instead, for this injury can easily be
treated. The cause of your shoulder pain is that the bursa
sac in the shoulder is mildly irritated and swollen. The
pain is felt in the shoulder and upper arm, usually only
when you lift your arm above shoulder height.

The anatomy of the shoulder bursa is described under
acute bursitis and you can find it on p. 156.

HOW AND WHY

A female friend of mine in her midthirties told me she had
been plagued with arthritis for five years. Sometimes
she'd have intense aching in one or both of her shoulders
and would grow frustrated and irritable when nothing re-

lieved it. Other times the ache bothered her only when she took off pullovers or reached up to high shelves. She never knew when she'd grow worse or how long she'd be in pain. Many, many medications and diets later, I brought her to a physician I work with, and she was surprised to learn that she didn't have arthritis. She had been suffering from chronic bursitis, and hers was an unusual case because it was in both shoulders rather than just one.

Chronic bursitis is as different from acute bursitis as fire is from ice. It is not horribly painful, but can last for years. It generally comes on for no apparent reason and can stay anywhere from a few months to ten years if it goes untreated. No one really knows what causes it or why it doesn't just go away.

DIAGNOSTIC VERIFICATION

Test

Stand with your arms at your sides and slowly lift your painful arm out from your side. As your arm approaches shoulder height there should be pain. Now continue to raise your arm until it is straight up. The pain should diminish quickly as you leave shoulder height and should not hurt the rest of the way up, though it may hurt when the arm is straight up. What is occurring is that the bursa gets pinched when your arm is near shoulder height. Chronic bursitis is a little complicated to evaluate yourself, because this same pain pattern occurs in three other injuries, but in those injuries it's only one of many symptoms. In this injury it's the primary indicator.

TREATMENT CHOICES

Medical Treatment

INJECTION: The only known effective treatment is one or two corticosteroid injections. My friend had a cortisone injection along with a local anaesthetic in both shoulders and was delighted when she could lift her arms without pain only two minutes later. It was explained that when the anaesthetic wore off in an hour she would again have pain for a few days until the medicine took effect. Five days later her five-year ordeal ended and she has been free of pain for over a year now. Massage, manipulation, and exercise do not help this condition and in fact can often make it worse.

Rehabilitation
After you feel no pain, begin the Weighted Arm Circle, p. 272. Do this exercise for a month.

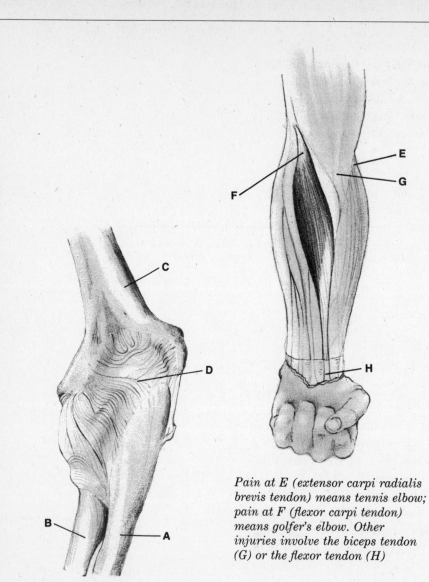

Pain at E (extensor carpi radialis brevis tendon) means tennis elbow; pain at F (flexor carpi tendon) means golfer's elbow. Other injuries involve the biceps tendon (G) or the flexor tendon (H)

The elbow joint, showing the ulna (A), the radius (B), the humerus (C), and the elbow-joint capsule (D)

The extensor tendon attachment (J), site of tennis elbow, and the lower extensor tendon attachment (I)

9

The Elbow

The most common use for an elbow is to prop up a tired head, in the pose immortalized by Rodin's *The Thinker*. It is such an inconspicuous part of the body that we rarely notice it unless something goes wrong. In this section we'll discuss the three most common elbow injuries, for they account for most of the pain in this area.

Three bones come together to form the elbow joint: two from the forearm (A and B) and one from the upper arm (C). If you have trouble fully bending or straightening your elbow, and it aches inside, then the irritation is in your elbow joint (D). If, however, your pain is on the outside (E) or the inside (F), you have tennis or golfer's elbow.

Elbow injuries are most often in the tendons of the muscles that attach to the elbow and are usually not in the muscle or joint itself. The muscles that attach at the elbow control wrist and hand movements. These tendon strains often radiate pain down the forearm.

The muscle that hurts when you have tennis elbow runs from the back of the wrist to the outer elbow (I J). If you raise a hammer you are using this muscle. There is another muscle that begins at the inner elbow and goes to the front of the wrist (FH), and this is the one that hurts when you have golfer's elbow. If you strike with a hammer you are using this muscle. These two tendon-muscle units control the movement of the wrist.

There are many other muscles of the forearm that can be strained, but these two injuries are the ones that cause the most troublesome problems. If you have a pain right in the front of the elbow in the midline at point G and it hurts here when you lift things or use a screwdriver, see biceps strain (p. 153); you have probably injured the lower tendon of the biceps muscle.

Be sure to read the whole Rehabilitation chapter, so you know how to use the exercises given later.

Tennis Elbow

WHAT IS IT?

If you are not a tennis player and you're relieved to think that this injury couldn't possible affect you, you're wrong. Tennis elbow earned its name because it has plagued some fine tennis players, but the vast majority of people who have this injury have never picked up a tennis racket. Tennis elbow means a slightly torn tendon near the elbow. It hurts at the outside of the elbow and at times the pain extends into the forearm as far as the wrist. To locate the exact spot, lean sideways against a wall and bend your arm as though you were going to shake hands with someone. Push your elbow against the wall. The knobby bone you feel is the place where the injured tendon attaches to the elbow. This is the place most commonly injured. The muscle-tendon unit extends down to the wrist at the back of your hand. Occasionally, you can be injured at other places along this unit. That's why the pain is sometimes felt all along the forearm.

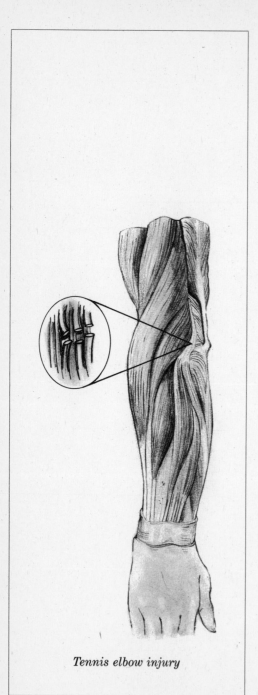

Tennis elbow injury

HOW AND WHY

This bothersome and often long-term injury is extremely common. It regularly attacks people who lift heavy objects, scrub floors, wait tables, and pour endless pots of coffee, and it frequently plagues racquet-sport fans. When racquet enthusiasts get tennis elbow it's usually because they haven't warmed up properly or because poor form caused unnecessary strain to the elbow.

In the beginning, tennis elbow is hardly discernible. After about two weeks the pain noticeably increases. It can get so bad that you drop things because of the sudden pain you feel.

Tennis elbow is complicated by reinjury: many racquet-sport players refuse to stop their activities because, when they are warmed up and playing, the pain diminishes—but it only reappears with more force later.

This tendon tears in a V shape, which makes healing quite difficult. Since the tear is wider at the top than at the bottom, it heals more quickly at the narrower bottom of the V (see diagram). At the top of the tear the new tissue has a greater distance to span and is therefore weaker. This uneven healing makes you feel better before the tendon is really knitted together, so it's easy to reinjure it and cause troublesome scar tissue.

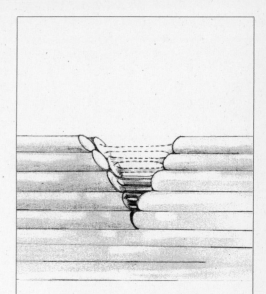

Tennis elbow's V-shape tear

DIAGNOSTIC VERIFICATION

Test

Stretch your arm out in front of you (see next page), making sure your elbow is straight, and bend your wrist as far as it will go, as if you were a traffic cop saying "Stop." It's easiest if you support the arm on a table or other chest-height object, as shown. Now place your other hand on the back of the extended hand and try to force the wrist down, as you strongly resist with the injured arm. If you have tennis elbow, this will reproduce your pain.

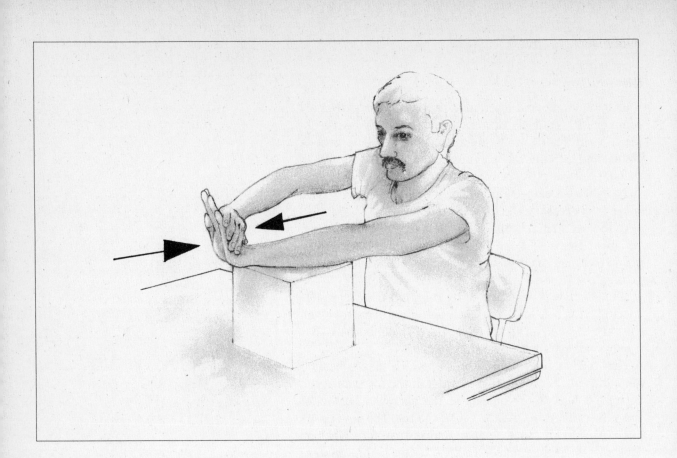

TREATMENT CHOICES

Self-Treatment

Self-treatment takes patience. You can use the ice treatment if you stop all strenuous activity for four to six weeks. Use the ice in conjunction with the Wrist Lift exercise, p. 270. In between icings you should hold a three- to five-pound weight in your hand. Raise and lower your wrist, working that muscle-tendon unit. Work up to ten or twelve pounds over a few weeks. Increase the weight only if it causes no pain. But be forewarned—you need to rest your elbow from athletic activity for two weeks after it feels completely fine. If this doesn't work, get some medical treatment. If it doesn't heal by itself within six to eight weeks with rest and ice, it may take anywhere from six months to a year to heal itself. In persons over sixty, healing has been known to take up to two years.

Medical Treatment

1. DEEP MASSAGE AND DEEP FRICTIONING: A combination of deep massage to the forearm to help circulation, and deep friction to break up the scar tissue, is often an effective treatment for tennis elbow. It is, however, a somewhat painful treatment.

2. INJECTION: Corticosteroid injection is an effective treatment only if the precise area of injury has been identified and injected thoroughly. If this has not occurred the pain will return. It is sometimes important to get several injections to stop the inflammation if part of the inflamed area was missed on the first injection. A week's rest should follow the injection, and then a period of strength building for a week or two until activity is resumed. If you have one weak muscle surrounded by many strong ones, the weak one will not be able to pull its weight and can become injured again easily. Proliferant injection is often a more effective treatment with a stubborn or long-standing tennis elbow. It helps to strengthen the tendon but may take a few more weeks to do its job of making you feel well again.

Rehabilitation
See the Wrist Lift, p. 270.

Inner Elbow Pain

(Golfer's Elbow)

WHAT IS IT?

If you are a really thorough pot scrubber who is at war with any black pot stains, you may scrub your way into this injury. Or, if you are an avid golfer or weight lifter who tends to overdo it, you can also end up injuring your inner elbows. To locate the source of this tendon strain, press your elbows into your sides, squeezing yourself as hard as you can. The injured tendon is attached to the

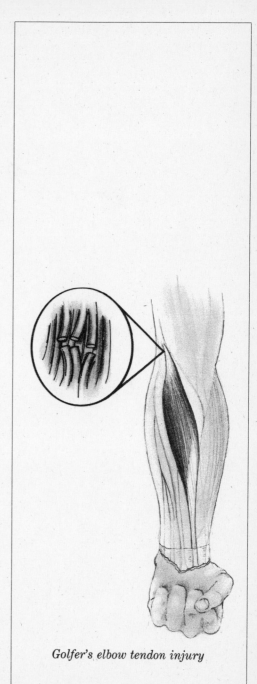

Golfer's elbow tendon injury

bone you feel squeezing your rib. The tendon is usually strained and painful where it attaches to the bone, but it can also be injured farther down the muscle-tendon unit. The more severe the injury, the more the pain radiates from the elbow to the wrist.

HOW AND WHY

It's hard to remember what you did to get golfer's elbow because the pain usually starts several days after the strain occurred, and almost any activity that uses a lot of forehand motion *can* give you this injury.

Golfer's elbow can stay a month or hang on for a year, depending on how well or poorly the strained fibers heal. If you keep repeating the activity that caused the strain originally, scarring may occur and prolong healing time.

DIAGNOSTIC VERIFICATION

Test
Sit at a table and extend your injured arm, palm up straight out in front of you, supporting your forearm with a book or something solid. Now bend the wrist of your injured arm, kept straight toward your face, and hold it there strongly. With your free hand make a fist and forcefully push it into the hand that is bent. Hold this isometric position for a few seconds. If this produces your pain at the inner elbow or slightly into your forearm, you have this injury.

TREATMENT CHOICES

Self-Treatment
If this injury is recent, it usually responds to ice treatment combined with the Wrist Bend exercise (p. 270) with light weights in a few weeks. With your palm up, hold a three- to five-pound weight in your hand and curl your hand up toward your face. Increase to ten to twelve pounds over several weeks only increasing the weight if it doesn't

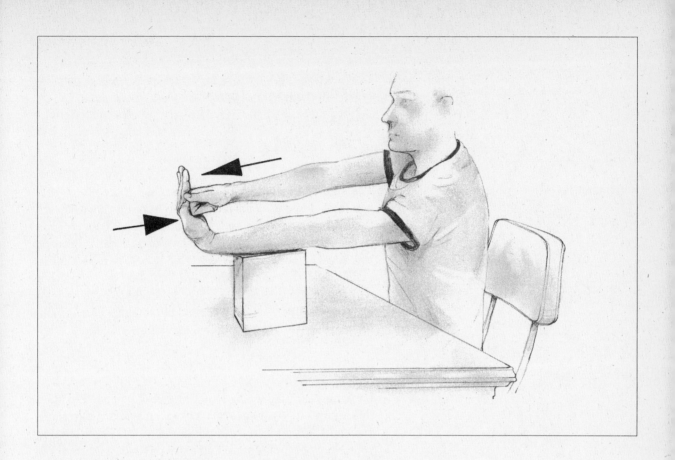

cause pain. Be sure to limit your activities, especially those that cause pain, until you are completely well.

Medical Treatment
1. DEEP FRICTIONING AND DEEP MASSAGE: A combination of these treatments is very effective because the tendon and muscle unit are easily accessible. This treatment usually takes from four to six weeks.
2. INJECTION: Corticosteroid injections are effective if all the strained fibers are thoroughly injected. This may take two or three visits. In long-standing, chronic injuries proliferant injections are often necessary to strengthen the tendon.

Rehabilitation
See the Wrist Bend, p. 270.

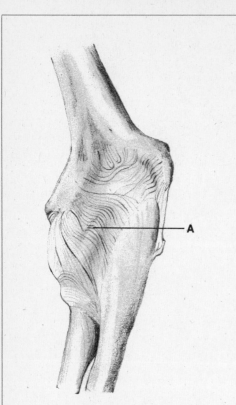

The elbow joint

Stiff Aching Elbow
(Traumatic Arthritis of the Elbow)

WHAT IS IT?

The sign of this injury is a deep aching in the elbow that you can't pinpoint. This pain usually spreads down toward the hand but can also go a little above the elbow. A joint (A) is actually a space between two bones that is encased by thousands of fibers. Within this space there is a lubricating fluid that allows the bones to slide on each other without friction. When you have injured your elbow joint many of the fibers dry and shrink, making movement painful because you are pulling and stretching the fibers.

HOW AND WHY

Banging your elbow into something is all you need to start this injury off. Over several weeks your pain usually worsens and the simple act of fully bending and straightening your elbow becomes more and more difficult. This injury is enigmatic. You can get it from throwing a ball for too many hours or after something as sedentary as reading a newspaper. All of which is to say we don't know what starts it.

DIAGNOSTIC VERIFICATION

When you have this injury you have more trouble fully bending your elbow than fully straightening it.

Test 1
Touch your shoulder with the hand of your injured elbow. Then using your other hand, press down further on the back of the wrist. If you have this injury, either you won't have been able to touch your shoulder or doing this test will cause pain.

Test 2

Now try to straighten your elbow all the way and again
either this will be too painful to do or doing it will cause
you pain.

TREATMENT CHOICES

Self-Treatment

You can buy an apparatus called a collar-and-cuff bandage
at a surgical-supply store. To use it, you bend your elbow
as far as you possibly can and then put on the bandage,
which fixes it in this position. Hold your elbow in this position for about two weeks, wearing the bandage constantly.
Every few days adjust the bandage to allow for gradual
straightening of the elbow. After six weeks you can gradu-
ate to a sling. Within two to three months you are better.
If this sounds horrid, it is. Happily, there is a much faster
treatment.

Medical Treatment

Two corticosteroid injections into the elbow joint given a
week apart eliminate this injury in two weeks. During this
recovery time you may use a sling for three or four days.
In mild cases one injection usually does the trick.

Massage, exercise, or stretching of the joint should be
avoided, as they make the injury worse.

10

The Thigh and Hip

The thigh is the muscular powerhouse of your body. Through it runs the toughest and longest bone that you've got—the femur. The four muscles of the front thigh are the strongest thigh muscles. You use them to kick, to run, and to walk. They are often collectively referred to as the quads, short for quadriceps. When they are injured it is rarely in the midsection of the thigh; usually strain occurs at the very top of the thigh, or where they attach to the knee just above the kneecap, p. 86.

The group of muscles on the inner part of the thigh is called the adductors (A, B, C, and D). They draw the legs together and stabilize your legs while you walk. The adductors are frequently injured near the groin and lower in the thigh. There is one small but strong muscle at the outer top thigh (E) that has a long tendon (F) that runs down to the outer knee. Lately injury to this muscle has been seen more often, owing to the popularity of long-distance running.

In the back thigh are the hamstrings which help you walk, run, climb, and stand. There are three of them (1, 2,

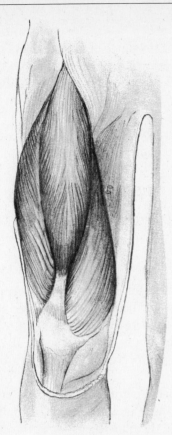

Front thigh muscles—the quadriceps

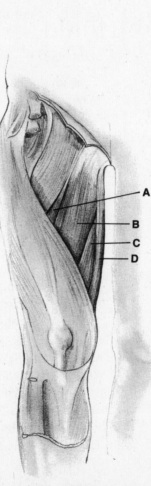

The adductors

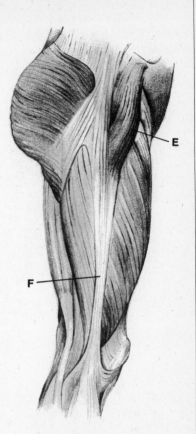

The tensor fascia lata muscle (E) and its tendon (F)

The hamstrings

Rectus femoris injury, showing the muscle (A) and the tendon (B)

and 3). They run from under the buttock to the back of the knee, moving outward and attaching below the knee. Injuries behind and below the knee were covered in the knee section, p. 99. Here we discuss tears of the mid- and upper hamstring.

Before doing any of the rehabilitative exercises, read through the Rehabilitation chapter that precedes them.

Front Hip or Front Thigh Pain
(Rectus Femoris Tendinitis, or Muscle Tear)

WHAT IS IT?

This injury is a real nemesis for dancers and runners. Where you hurt will depend on whether you've injured the tendon (B) or the muscles (A). If your pain is in the front of the hip, you've strained the fibers of the tendon. If it's lower down in the front thigh, you've strained or torn the muscle fibers.

The muscle-tendon unit usually injured is called the rectus femoris. This muscle is the longest and strongest muscle of the four that comprise the quadriceps—it is the one that helps you lift the thigh. The other three only help you straighten the knee.

HOW AND WHY

This is one of the few injuries people get from stretching their front thighs in an attempt to counteract the strain of hard running; they end up stretching their tendons out, weakening the fibers, and making them more vulnerable to injuries. Because this weakening is a slow process, you can overstretch for years before getting this injury.*

Climbing or hiking down steep hills or mountains, especially where the terrain is gravelly or slippery, can cause

*However, if you stretch properly, feeling the pull in the muscle and not the tendon, this weakening will not occur. See *Sports Without Pain*.

the front thigh to contract suddenly and become injured. What happens is this: as you start to slip or fall, the front thigh grabs so severely that it causes either a massive tear throughout the muscle or a tear in the tendon. I got this injury in a very interesting way—slipping and sliding down a gravelly mountain running from a snake. I never covered so much territory so fast.

In cases where the tear is severe, walking becomes painfully difficult and running impossible. In milder cases, walking feels all right, but lifting the leg straight up in front or doing a single leg lift from a lying-down position hurts.

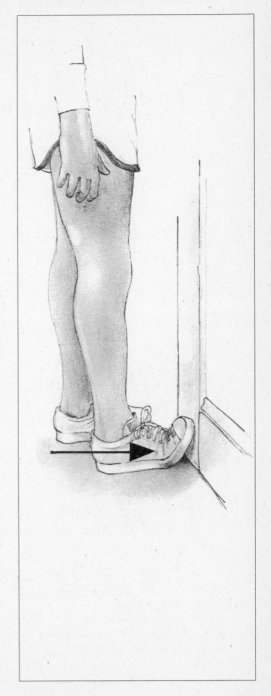

DIAGNOSTIC VERIFICATION

Test
Wearing shoes, stand about six inches away from a wall. With the legs straight, place the toe of your injured foot against the wall. Now press your toe straight into the wall as hard as you can without bending the knee. If you have a rectus femoris tear, this should hurt. In addition, if you grab hold of your foot and bring your heel to your buttock, as if trying to stretch the thigh, this may cause pain. If the pain is felt deep at the front of the hip, it might be arthritis of the hip, which is sometimes helped by injection.

TREATMENT CHOICES

Self-Treatment
If you rest and use the ice treatment along with the Thigh Lift (p. 268), healing can take anywhere from a week or two to six or eight weeks, depending on how badly you've torn the muscle. If you've torn the tendon, ice may not work because the tendon is too deep. Avoid all activity that causes pain, but do try to start moving it gently as soon as you can do so without pain.

Medical Treatment
1. DEEP FRICTIONING: For injuries to the tendon at the top of the thigh, deep frictioning is effective, al-

though somewhat painful. This area is commonly sensitive and needs the attention of a skilled therapist. Because the tendon is so deep and lies underneath some others, the thigh must sometimes be bent at a 90° angle in order to get at it.

2. DEEP MASSAGE: This procedure is therapeutic for tears in the muscle. It moves the blood through the injured area and promotes healing.

3. INJECTION: A corticosteroid injection is a fast and effective way to deal with injury to the tendon. Corticosteroids can help prevent or eliminate extensive unwanted scar tissue from forming in massive tearing throughout the front thigh muscle.

Rehabilitation

See the first three Knee and Thigh exercises, p. 268 and p. 269.

Inner Thigh and Groin Pain
(Adductor Tendinitis)

WHAT IS IT?

If you are an athlete, a dancer, or a gymnast, a pulled groin muscle can be a tenacious, enduring injury. With this injury you feel pain in your inner-upper thigh. If the pain is only in this area, you've injured the tendon (X) of one of the four adductor muscles (A, B, C, or D). If the pain is toward the mid-thigh, you've injured the fibers of the muscle (Y). If you feel pain in both places, you are unfortunate enough to have injured both the tendon and the muscle.

The adductor muscles draw your legs together, help stabilize your legs in walking or running, and work especially hard when you are doing side-to-side movements. The adductors are anchored into the pubic bone at the top of the thigh and run to the mid-thigh or the inside of the knee.

Injured adductor tendons (Y), showing the adductor brevis (A), the adductor longus (B), the adductor magnus (C), the gracilus (D), and the adductor tendons (X)

HOW AND WHY

This injury rarely has dramatic causes, such as a fall or blow. It typically occurs as a result of forced stretching or vigorous activity without a good warm-up, especially where quick side-to-side movement is required, as in tennis, racquetball, squash, and basketball. In the worst cases even walking hurts, but more commonly, you feel pain only during vigorous activity or when stretching the inner-thigh muscles. If treated properly, this injury can be gone in two to three weeks, but if ignored, it can plague you for years.

DIAGNOSTIC VERIFICATION

Test

Sit on the floor with your legs out in front of you. Place a ball between your knees and try to squeeze your knees together as hard as you can. That should reproduce your pain. Another way to test it is to sit on the floor with your legs spread wide apart and bring your chest toward the floor. This stretches the inner thigh and may also cause pain. You don't need to know which muscle or tendon is injured. If you can place your finger directly on the painful spot during the test you'll know where treatment has to be given. If the pain is pretty severe, especially in the groin area, see a doctor for an X ray. Young people in their teens sometimes fracture part of the lower pelvis, which is as yet not fully changed from cartilage to bone. This can prove serious if not attended to properly; therefore, it's best to check it out even though it's relatively rare.

TREATMENT CHOICES

Self-Treatment

If you catch this injury, early self-treatment can be quite effective. Rest and absolutely no stretching are essential in the early phase of this injury. Ice treatment should be started along with the Thigh Squeeze exercise, p. 269, as soon as possible. As the condition improves, you can participate in athletic activity, provided there is no pain during or after. If you experience pain, *Stop*. It means you're not ready yet. Of course, begin with some moderate activity, such as easy jogging, swimming, or strength exercises on the floor; not basketball or running ten miles. Pull back if you begin to feel pain again, and go a bit slower. After you have felt no pain for two weeks' time, begin stretching very gently.

Medical Treatment

1. DEEP FRICTIONING AND DEEP MASSAGE: These treatments are usually extremely helpful in cutting down your healing time. If the injury has been with you for a long time, there is some poorly formed scar tissue there, and deep friction would be the best method to pursue.
2. INJECTION: Corticosteroid injections are effective in the case of new injuries as well as in long-standing stubborn ones.

Rehabilitation

See the Thigh Squeeze (p. 269), and try Knee Extensions with the leg turned out a little, which gets the inner thigh muscles to work more.

Diagonal Pain Across the Inner Thigh

(Sartorius Tear)

WHAT IS IT?

Sartorius means the "tailor's" muscle—in olden times tailors sat cross-legged on the floor, stretching that muscle. In this injury some fibers in the muscle-tendon unit (A) become strained or torn. The most common place for the tearing to occur is where the tendon joins the muscle: two to four inches below the hip bone and slightly toward the inside of the thigh (B).

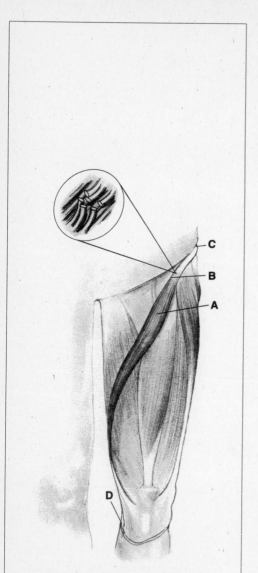

Injured sartorius muscle-tendon unit, showing the muscle (A), the upper tendon attachment (C), and the lower tendon attachment (D). The most frequent injury site is at B.

Pain is generally limited to a small segment of the top of the thigh, but in cases where the injury is severe, pain can encompass a large area extending down the muscle.

The sartorius muscle begins at the bony part of the front of the hip (C), which is prominent in skinny people. It then runs diagonally across the thigh and attaches below the inner side of the knee (D). This muscle helps you lift your leg up and out to the side, and also helps you lift your leg to the front when it is turned out, as a dancer might do.

HOW AND WHY

Usually this injury comes on rather suddenly—when, for example, you try to do a spectacular split. It can also be caused by overworking the muscle. This injury occurs mostly to dancers or gymnasts who do much of their training with their legs in a turned-out position.

DIAGNOSTIC VERIFICATION

It can be difficult to distinguish this injury from an adductor tear (p. 180) or a rectus femoris tear (p. 178) because the muscles overlap. Be sure to read about those injuries and do the diagnostic verification tests for them as well.

Test

Sit on the floor and place the soles of your feet together with your legs turned out as shown on the next page. Then let the good leg slide forward. Place your hand on the inner surface of the knee of the injured leg, and try to raise your knee to the ceiling while resisting with the force of your arm and hand. If you have this injury, that should cause you pain or discomfort. It should help you find its precise location as well.

TREATMENT CHOICES

Self-Treatment

With rest and ice treatments done along with Knee Extensions, p. 268, healing may take three to six weeks. Treat-

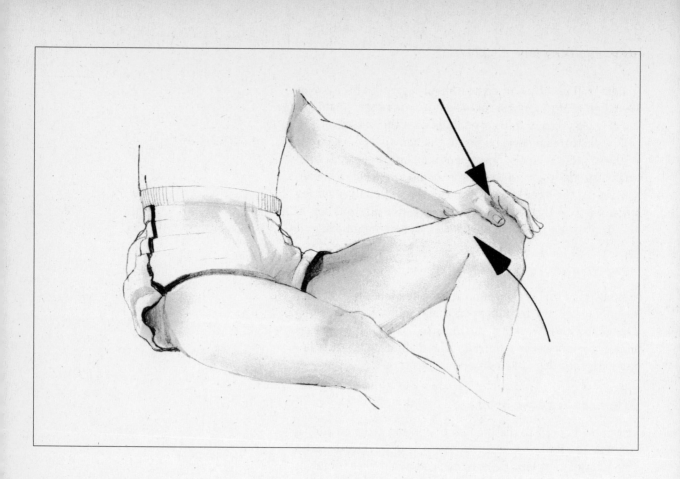

ing this injury yourself takes lots of patience. Take your
time—if you keep using the leg, you may reinjure the area
and chronic, painful scar tissue may form.

Medical Treatment
1. DEEP FRICTIONING AND DEEP MASSAGE: Either of these
   techniques can effect healing within just a week or
   two.
2. INJECTION: Since healing is usually quite easy, corticosteroid injections are not recommended unless the
   tearing has become chronic. In such cases, a well-
   placed injection is quite effective.

Rehabilitation
See the first three Knee and Thigh exercises, pp. 268–69.

Pulled Hamstring

WHAT IS IT?

Those little strings behind your knee have long Latin names, but we'll skip them. Those are your hamstrings. "Pulled hamstring" is a term often used to describe pain in the back of the thigh. What it really means is that some fibers—belonging to either a hamstring muscle or tendon—are strained or torn. The pain can be felt anywhere along the back of the thigh or up near the lower part of the buttock.

There are three hamstrings (1, 2, and 3), all beginning at the base of the buttock—the bone you sit on. These long muscles of the back thigh span two joints: the hip and the knee. They help you run, jump, and climb upstairs. (1) and (2) control the inner half of the back thigh. They attach just below the front of the knee. (3) covers the outer half of the back thigh and attaches to the outside of the knee. Injuries to any part of the hamstring near the knee joint can easily be mistaken for problems of the knee itself.

HOW AND WHY

Suddenly you've got it—pain in the back of the thigh. Hamstring injuries usually occur without warning. Running hurts, climbing stairs may be painful, and stretching is the worst.

If you hurt in the back of your thigh when using those muscles there's a 90 percent chance that you have a pulled hamstring because they are the only things back there. A painful sensation in the middle of the back thigh means that muscle fibers are torn. Pain high up near the bottom of the buttock means that the tendon attaching the hamstring to the sit bone is affected. Injuries to the muscle often heal quickly because of the excellent blood supply that pumps through continuously, but they can heal with poor

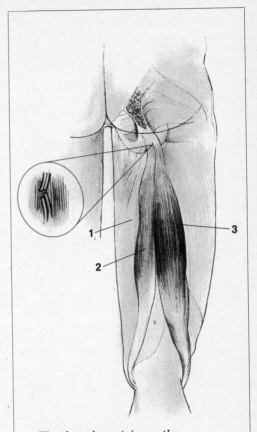

The three hamstrings—the semimembranosis (1), the semitendinosis (2), and the biceps femoris (3)—showing a tear at the upper attachment

scar-tissue formation and become a chronic problem. Hamstring tendon tears heal more slowly and need more care. The initial injury usually occurs while stretching or running—especially when there has been no prior warm-up. The cold muscle resists stress when tension is suddenly placed on it, and something gives. This is also likely to happen if the muscle is fatigued.

When you feel pain deep within your back thigh, especially after prolonged sitting, it could be referred pain from a lower-back injury. To be sure, check pages 250, 241, and 245 to differentiate the two.

A hamstring injury can go on for months if not treated properly. A young athlete once came to me with a chronic hamstring problem and said, "I've been stretching my hamstrings religiously—every day for seven months. I can't understand why it's not better." The reason he wasn't getting better was this daily stretching. It was tearing apart the new young tissue that was trying to form, and wasn't allowing the fibers time to heal and become strong. It was creating poorly formed scar tissue, causing mini-reinjuries. His original injury could have healed up and disappeared with rest—but instead it became chronic because of premature activity.

DIAGNOSTIC VERIFICATION

Test
Face a chair, place the heel of your foot on it, and slowly stretch forward. If this reproduces your pain, one of your hamstrings is probably injured. As you stretch forward, try to locate the exact spot as precisely as you can. This will help you know where to direct your therapy. Also try the test on p. 101.

TREATMENT CHOICES

Self-Treatment
It's important to avoid activities that create pain whenever possible. Do not stretch until you are better, and then

go gently at first. Follow the ice treatment for as long as you can stand it. During the ice treatment and throughout the day, bend the knee of your injured leg by bringing the foot to your opposite knee ten to fifteen times while in a standing position. This will help to prevent the formation of unwanted scar tissue.

The entire healing process should take between a week and six weeks, depending upon how severe the injury. If the above treatment does not seem to be helping and you want to speed your recovery, seek out one of the medical treatments described below. They are usually faster than doing it yourself.

Medical Treatment
1. DEEP FRICTIONING AND DEEP MASSAGE: These treatments are very effective for increasing circulation and inhibiting poor scar tissue from developing.
2. INJECTION: Corticosteroid injections are usually the fastest treatment, although most people prefer not to go the route of injections. In cases of long-standing hamstring pain, a combination of local anaesthetic and corticosteroid is often the *only* means of effective treatment, because scar tissue from chronic retearing has become so prevalent.

Rehabilitation
See Hamstring Strengtheners, p. 269.

Severe Bruising of the Thigh
(Hematoma)

WHAT IS IT?

I've included this injury under the thigh, although it can occur at other spots in the body as well. A hematoma looks like a huge bruise. It can be red, purple, or black and blue, and swollen like a grapefruit. It most frequently happens as a result of a kick or some type of collision in contact sports, roller skating, or a fall down the stairs. Blood vessels within the body break open and blood pours into the surrounding area under the skin. The body then closes off these broken vessels, but the blood that has escaped is trapped where it is. It can be very painful, and usually encompasses a large area—as much as six inches in diameter.

WHERE

A hematoma can occur anywhere in the body but is most frequently found in the front, outside, or back of the thigh, the shin, or the calf. The swelling is most prominent when it occurs at the outer thigh.

TREATMENT CHOICES

Self-Treatment

If the swelling is slight, ice treatment and rest for five to ten days will take care of it. If it is very swollen or painful, see a doctor as soon as you can. If the blood that is trapped between and within the muscles should remain there and not be reabsorbed by the body, calcium can form within the muscle tissue, causing the muscle to stiffen up permanently.

Medical Treatment

A corticosteroid injection of the entire area of the hematoma will diminish the pain quickly after the pooled blood is removed through a needle. Injection of corticosteroid will then reduce the chances of getting calcium deposits in the bruised muscle.

Pain at the Outer Hip
(Trochanteric Bursitis)

WHAT IS IT?

This is a mean, nasty little injury, but it can be cleared up in a snap. It is an irritation/inflammation of the bursa that lies between the upper thigh bone and the skin. To find the location of the bursa just lie on the floor on your side. The bursa covers the bone you feel sticking into the floor. The pain is felt near the skin surface of the outermost point of the hip (A). This part of the upper thigh bone is called the greater trochanter, which is where the bursa gets its name.

HOW AND WHY

What really causes this irritation is unknown. Pain in this bursa often appears for no apparent reason, though sometimes a fall might precipitate it. In severe but rare cases the pain may travel down the outer thigh.

DIAGNOSTIC VERIFICATION

Test
Lie on a wooden floor or hard surface on the painful side. This should cause an increase in your pain.

TREATMENT CHOICES

Medical Treatment
The only effective treatment known is corticosteroid injection directly into the bursa. Total relief usually comes within several days of this treatment.

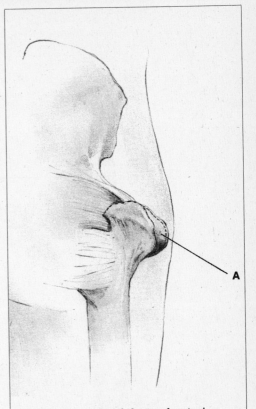

Inflammation of the trochanteric bursa

11
The Lower Leg

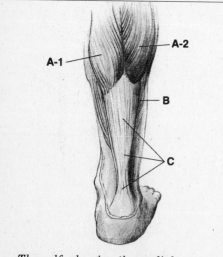

The calf, showing the medial gastrocnemius (A-1), the lateral gastrocnemius (A-2), the soleus (B), and the Achilles tendon (C)

The lower leg—which can be plagued by broken bones, shin splints, Achilles tendon injuries, and cramps that wake you in the middle of the night—comprises the shin and the calf.

The calf has only two important muscles. The one you feel when you touch your calf is called the gastrocnemius. This muscle has two halves: one toward the inside (A-1) and one toward the outside of the calf (A-2). Beneath it lies the soleus muscle (B), which holds the real strength and power in the calf. These muscles help you walk, run, and rise up on your toes. They are both attached to the back of the heel by the Achilles tendon (C).

Now to the front of your lower leg, your shin. If you place your hand on the front of your lower leg and pull your toes toward your knee flexing your foot and ankle, you will see and feel the main shin muscle (D) pop out slightly. It starts below the knee, is about one and a half to two inches wide in the middle, and has a long tendon at its lower end that goes from above the front of the ankle to the inner instep (E).

190

You can't see or feel the other shin muscle easily because it's behind the shin bone deep in the middle of the lower leg. Its tendon wraps around the back of your inner ankle and also attaches on the inner instep. This shin muscle helps you hold your instep up, keeps your foot from wobbling on uneven surfaces, and works in all walking and running activities. When either of your shin muscles is injured it's referred to as "shin splints."

Severe Surface Calf Pain
(Gastrocnemius Strain or Muscle Tear)

WHAT IS IT?

Picture yourself walking around on the ball of your foot, unable to put your heel down—that's what happens if you have this injury. It's awkward and very painful. With this injury, there is a severe strain and tearing of the calf muscle fibers. The pain is felt near the middle of the calf and is perceived as occurring somewhere near the surface, rather than deep inside.

This calf muscle has two parts: an inner one (A-1) and an outer one (A-2). They begin at the back of the lower thigh and join together in one common tendon, the Achilles (C). These are important muscles for walking. They also help you rise up onto the balls of your feet—particularly with straight knees.

HOW AND WHY

The story I've most often heard from people with this injury goes like this: "I got this pain in my calf a week ago while I was playing ball. I just thought it would go away so I kept on playing. Now I can't put my heel down when I walk sometimes. It hurts too much."

Tearing in the middle or upper part of the muscle can also happen with a snap. People describe it like this: "It

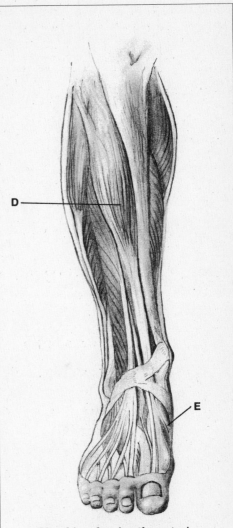

The shin, showing the anterior tibialis muscle (D) and the tendon attachment (E)

felt like somebody hit me with a racket across my calf, but when I turned to see, no one was there."

With this injury usually the fibers are torn only microscopically. Walking is uncomfortable and any greater exertion may cause pain. When pain is extreme, there can be a tear in the muscle that is so wide it leaves a half-inch gap. When this happens standing is excruciating—and the only way to walk is on the ball of the foot of your injured leg. But in most cases you can stand without pain—it's being more active that makes it hurt.

In chronic cases that have healed poorly, the injury gets alternately better and worse—the worst bouts of pain lasting as long as six months.

The causes of this type of tear are varied. Excess muscle tension in the lower legs, lack of a proper warm-up before workouts, or general fatigue in the legs, all combined with overexertion, are the most common contributing factors.

DIAGNOSTIC VERIFICATION

One sure sign of this injury is that you can't stand with your leg straight and your heel on the ground, and you can walk relatively comfortably only on the ball of your foot. If you sit down, you can flex your foot much better with your knee bent than you can with it straight. If the pain is so bad that you can't put your heel down, don't do the following test. (Only do it if your pain is moderate.)

Test

Stand with your feet parallel and knees straight. Rise way up on your half toe (the ball of your foot). If you feel no pain, do the same test standing only on the injured leg. If you have a tear of the gastrocnemius muscle, it should be painful to rise up with your knee straight. (The reason it's more comfortable to *walk* on the ball of your foot is that you are simultaneously bending the knee and relaxing your injured calf muscle. In the test you are *standing* with knees straight, working the muscle.) If this doesn't produce pain, see the section on soleus strains (p. 194).

(p. 194)

TREATMENT CHOICES

Self-Treatment

If you choose to treat this yourself, be *very* careful. Be sure not to jump into full activity too soon. Get some felt or moleskin and make a thick pad to fit in the heel of your shoe. It should be thick enough so that you can stand and walk without any pain. You may want to build up the other foot equally so that you don't feel lopsided, and you may need to build it up as much as an inch or an inch and a half, depending on the extent of your injury. Keep going till you feel comfortable. You can also opt to wear high-heeled shoes instead. Raising the heel takes the pressure off of the torn muscle.

Do the ice treatment, taking frequent breaks, alternately flexing and pointing your foot with the knee *slightly* bent. Continue doing this pointing and flexing throughout the day while in a sitting position. Do it with the knee bent at first, the goal being to do this exercise with the leg almost straight within a week or so. Do not attempt it if it produces pain.

When the calf is feeling better, do the rehabilitative exercises shown on p. 266 two or three times a day. It's important to keep moving so that scar tissue doesn't form where it shouldn't. Movement during healing helps cut down on scar tissue and helps the muscle stay flexible.

Medical Treatment
1. DEEP FRICTIONING AND DEEP MASSAGE: In moderate cases this treatment, combined with the measures explained above, will make the healing faster and help ensure the least scar-tissue formation. But in severe cases of a substantial tear, a doctor should be seen and treatments should not commence until a few days after the injury.
2. INJECTION: Injections of corticosteroids are effective

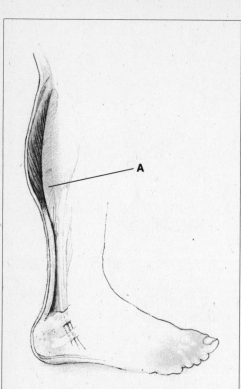

The soleus muscle (A)

in treating this injury, particularly if it has been a long-standing problem.

Rehabilitation

When you are fully recovered, start the Heel Raises exercise (p. 266). Start very slowly and build gradually to forty or fifty repetitions with a rest every ten.

Deep Calf Pain

(Soleus Strain or Muscle Tear)

WHAT IS IT?

If you stay in bed a lot you'll never get this injury—you have to do a lot of strenuous running or dancing to be vulnerable to it. If you strain or tear your soleus, pain is felt deep in the calf, usually in the upper part, toward the knee. Discomfort can be felt in one spot or over a broad area, because when you injure the soleus muscle (A) many small fibers are torn and inflamed.

The soleus is the largest, strongest calf muscle and lies underneath the gastrocnemius muscle, which was discussed on p. 191. The soleus starts at the top of the calf and attaches to the Achilles tendon at the bottom.

HOW AND WHY

There's a run on this injury after marathons, especially after the Boston Marathon, where the course goes uphill. When you run uphill you are forced to bend your knees more than usual and that puts a lot of stress on the soleus muscle. This same kind of stress is experienced if you do a lot of high jumping and land badly.

You'll feel a dull, aching kind of pain during and directly after strenuous activity. This injury isn't as debilitating as many but still puts a stop to the strenuous activities you enjoy.

DIAGNOSTIC VERIFICATION

Test

Stand barefooted with your feet parallel. Bend your knees
as far as you can keeping your heels firmly on the floor and
your back erect. Now rise high onto the balls of your feet
several times while keeping your knees bent. If you have
injured your soleus muscle, this should cause a momentary
increase in pain. If the test doesn't work, try it again after
strenuous activity, when your leg is already aching. To increase the stress on the injured area you might need to do
the test only on the injured leg holding onto something for
support.

If this test does not produce an increase in pain, you
may have injured your other calf muscle and should check
p. 191.

TREATMENT CHOICES

Self-Treatment

Self-treatment requires as much patience as there is
strain. The larger the strain the longer the time. Ice treatment with bent-leg Heel Raises (see below) and rest are
sometimes effective but may take many months. The big
danger is returning to strenuous activity too soon without
slowly building up.

Medical Treatment

1. DEEP FRICTIONING COMBINED WITH DEEP MASSAGE: This is
   the best treatment for this injury because the injury
   is usually over a wide area. This treatment is very
   effective, although it can take from five to eight
   weeks for the injury to get better.
2. INJECTION: When the injury is felt in one localized spot
   injection of corticosteroids is effective.

Rehabilitation

Start slowly with Heel Raises (p. 266), but do them with
your knees bent slightly (three inches).

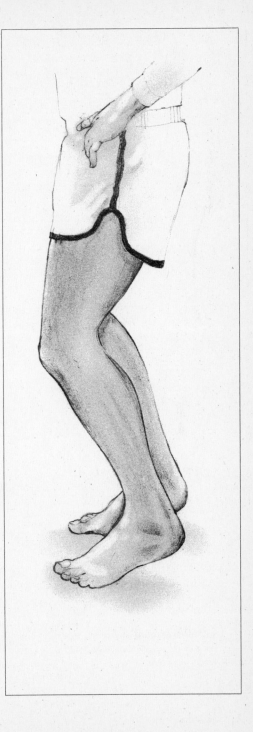

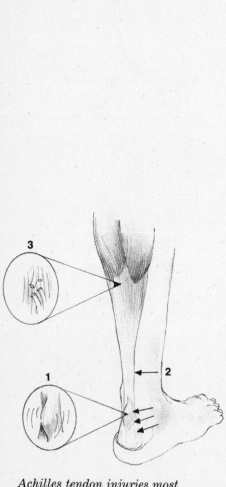

Achilles tendon injuries most frequently occur at points 1, 2, or 3

Pain in the Lower Calf or Behind the Ankle

(Achilles Tendinitis)

WHAT IS IT?

Tiptoeing discreetly and quietly in or out of the back door is almost impossible if you have Achilles tendinitis because it hurts too much. Runners and ballerinas are equally miserable with it. Often you feel this injury in more than one place. You may hurt just behind and above the heel, or an inch higher behind the ankle, or several inches up in the lower calf. The pain may vary too. It can range from a mild aching sensation to a severe throbbing pain. When you've injured the Achilles tendon, fibers can be torn or swollen or the thin, cellophanelike sheath that surrounds the tendon with nourishing fluid can be irritated.

The Achilles is one of your biggest and strongest tendons. Without it you could not walk. This tendon begins at the back of the heel and extends up to the middle of the calf. It connects all the calf muscles to the heel and controls the actions of pushing off in walking and running and rising on the balls of your feet. This tendon changes shape as it moves up the calf. Behind the heel and toward the midcalf the tendon is broad and flat, while in between these two places it's more rounded and ropelike.

HOW AND WHY

Your Achilles tendon doesn't like to be stretched, but for some reason people are convinced that stretching is good for it. Runners seem especially convinced of this and injure their Achilles tendon through poor stretching techniques. Folk dancers exhaust and strain it by jumping up and down on the balls of their feet for hours at a time, and ballet and modern dancers abuse this tendon by pointing their feet too hard. It's most frequently strained at points 1 and 2 (see illustration). Ballet and modern dancers frequently strain this tendon at the top of their heel 1 or 2, and runners and athletes generally injure it at points 2 or 3. In a moderate strain the fibers swell, causing discomfort, and the swelling can often be felt around the tendon at the back of the ankle. But the Achilles tendon has four surfaces—a front, a back, and two sides—and can be injured on any one or several of its surfaces. As a result you can feel pain in many places.

A severely injured Achilles hurts more and persists longer, because some of the fibers tear; in its worst form this injury rips the tendon completely in half, leaving you unable to walk. Another type of problem with the Achilles occurs when a granular material forms between the sheath and the tendon, causing a rubbing irritation to both; but we don't really know why this one happens.

DIAGNOSTIC VERIFICATION

Test

To test for this injury stand barefooted and rise high onto the balls of your feet. You may have to do this several times on both feet, or perhaps do it only on your injured leg, in order to reproduce the pain. If you feel pain only after strenuous activity, wait until then to do the test; if the Achilles is injured, your pain will momentarily increase. If you've had pain in the tendon and swelling for quite a while, you should see your doctor to check for gout.

TREATMENT CHOICES

Self-Treatment

This is a bear, a real tough one to treat yourself, unless your strain is very mild. If your pain comes and goes, be sure to seek professional help, because this is a sign that you need it. Ice treatment along with gentle pointing and flexing of the foot is helpful in mild strains. Wearing a shoe that has an inch heel takes the pressure off the tendon when you're walking, and this can help too. You can also build up the inside of your heel with several Dr. Scholl's

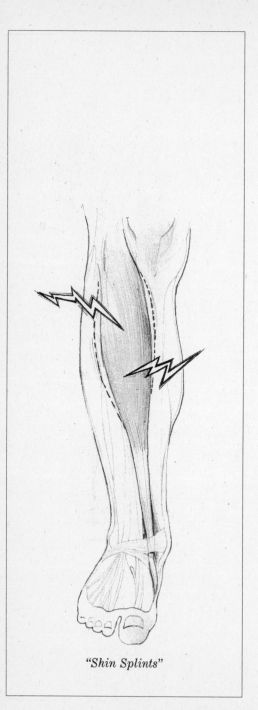

"Shin Splints"

heel pads to take the pressure off the tendon. It's important to avoid any activity that causes pain.

Medical Treatment
1. DEEP FRICTIONING AND DEEP MASSAGE: A combination of these treatments is often effective but can take up to six to eight weeks with two to three treatments per week. Unfortunately, this treatment can be fairly painful. It's important to remember that activity must be re-entered gradually or reinjury is likely.
2. INJECTION: Corticosteroid and proliferant injections have been used effectively in some of these injuries. The difficulty with this treatment is that the injured area is often so inflamed that it's hard to inject properly in a single visit.
3. SURGERY: In cases where the tendon has completely ruptured surgery is required.

Rehabilitation
Do Heel Raises, p. 266, when you are pain free.

"Shin Splints"
(Pain on Either Side of the Shin Bone)

WHAT IS IT?

You have a lot of trouble kicking people when you have this injury, and running up hills and jumping aren't fun either. This injury has been with us so long and is so common that it's acquired a totally nonsensical nickname, "shin splints." Splints have nothing to do with it. We are actually talking about two different injuries that have the same name. In both cases the muscle fibers swell and, in more severe cases, slightly tear. "Shin splints" create an aching pain that can be quite severe while running, jumping, and in bad cases even when walking. To make matters worse, you frequently get them in both legs at once.

One shin muscle, A, lies to the outside of your shin bone,

and when it hurts it is easy to feel and locate. The other is a little trickier, for it lies behind your shin bone. You can feel only the very edge of it if you press on the ridge at the inside of your shin bone, B. When you've injured that muscle you feel a dull, nagging pain on the inside of your lower leg.

HOW AND WHY

There has been a big run on this injury since runners have taken over the countryside because strenuous use combined with poor alignment in the foot—a dropping arch— is hard on weekend runners' shins. In everyday usage a foot-alignment problem wouldn't cause injury, but the extra stress of running or other intense athletics—dancing on a hard concrete floor, for example—can tip the balance. This long-term injury can drag on for years if not treated properly, and can last months even with good care. In addition, it can come and go unless preventive measures are taken. And if you don't take this problem seriously, it can develop into something more severe.

I remember a woman whose shins got sore running. Her husband's advice was not to baby herself and run through the pain, and unfortunately she listened to him. She ended up with multiple stress fractures of the shin bone. These fractures are actually hairline cracks of the bone, which are extremely painful. Here's what occurs: the shin muscles are supposed to absorb the shock of stress as you pound the pavement. When they are not strained or over-fatigued, they do this job very well. When they are strained the muscles quit, and if you continue to push beyond this point, the bone must take hundreds of pounds of stress on itself. This it can't do for more than a very brief time, and so it begins to develop cracks.

The woman in my story was pretty angry at her husband as he ran off each day while she nursed her leg back into shape. It took her months to build her leg back up to the point where she could begin to run again.

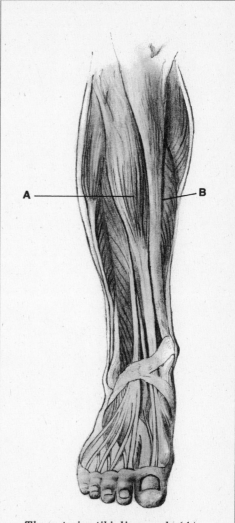

The anterior tibialis muscle (A) and the posterior tibialis muscle (B)

DIAGNOSTIC VERIFICATION

Test 1

If your pain is in the front part of your shin and slightly to the outside, at least one of the following two tests should reproduce your discomfort. The first one is simple. Wearing shoes, raise your toes off the floor and balance on your heels. Be sure to hold onto something so you don't fall. After doing this for a moment, severely strained shins will begin to hurt.

Test 2

For the next test sit in a chair and flex your foot by pulling your toes toward your knee. While keeping your foot flexed, place your hand over the top of your foot, and with your hand forcefully try to push your foot down while resisting in a flexed position. If this makes your shin hurt, you've got "shin splints."

Test 3

Here is a test for pain on the inner side of the shin. If you find that you are in pain only after an activity, do the test immediately following the activity. Otherwise this test may not reproduce your pain. Sit in a chair with your injured leg crossing over your other leg. Raise your foot toward the ceiling and hold it there no matter what. Now place your palm over the inner side of your big toe joint and press down as hard as you can. This should reproduce or increase your pain.

TREATMENT CHOICES

Self-Treatment

Self-treatment is possible only when fatigue is the major factor in your strain. In these cases rest and ice treatment done along with Ankle Flexion, p. 266, are effective. During the ice treatment, exercise by flexing and pointing your foot thirty to fifty times every fifteen minutes. If possible you should stop all the activities that are causing you pain.

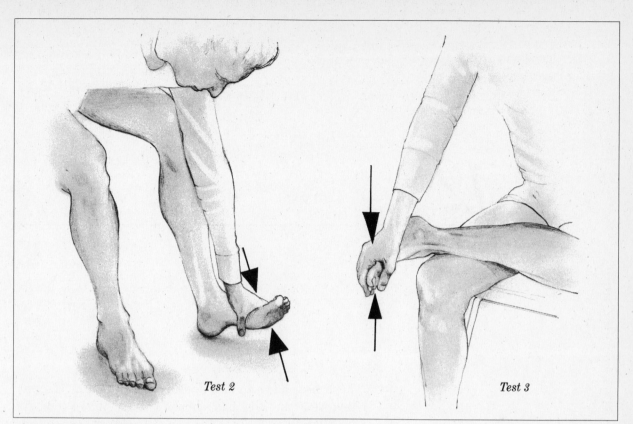

Test 2

Test 3

Medical Treatment

1. DEEP FRICTIONING AND DEEP MASSAGE: These treatments are most effective if you've injured the muscle on the outside of the shin bone. The other one, which is harder to reach, is helped only indirectly by the increase in general circulation.

2. ORTHOTICS: These are molded arch supports, which help to align the feet and take the unnecessary stress off the shin muscles. They are described in detail on p. 38 and must be purchased from a sports podiatrist. Orthotics combined with frictioning and deep massage are very effective.

3. INJECTION: You can use injections only when the affected area is very small; otherwise it's difficult to get it all.

Rehabilitation

See Heel Raises and Ankle Flexion, p. 266.

12

The Spine

"So, I bent down to pick up the newspaper and bam, my back went out." If I had a dime for every time I've heard the complaint "My back went out" I could retire. In fact, one out of every four people in the United States has had a back or neck problem at some time. Most back and neck problems relate to injuries to some part of the spine.

The spine is the supporting beam of our bodies; it gives us our form, and it houses and protects the spinal cord, the connecting link in our nervous system between our bodies and our brain. The spine is actually twenty-six separate bones that fit with puzzlelike intricacy; hundreds of small muscles and ligaments that move and provide the supporting links of the spine; discs, which cushion and separate the vertebrae; over forty-eight major nerves, which are the main terminals for the communication network between the nervous system and the rest of our body; and, finally, over seventy separate joints that determine the way we move our back and neck. When we consider the weblike complexity of the spine we can appreciate the difficulty in fully understanding it and evaluating what goes wrong.

BASIC STRUCTURES OF THE SPINE

The bones of your spine are called vertebrae: they are stacked one on top of the other, forming a long, thin, tapering column from top to bottom. The different shapes and sizes of the vertebrae allow for varying kinds of movement—for instance, your neck moves more freely than your midback because of the way the bones are constructed. There are seven thin vertebrae in the neck, twelve vertebrae in the midback, and five in the lower back.

At the bottom of your spine there are five vertebrae that fuse in early childhood into a triangular-shaped bone (the sacrum). The sacrum is a part of the spine; it joins the trunk to the legs and is held to the pelvis by a mass of important crisscrossing ligaments.

Between each of the bones of the spine lies a spongy cartilage called a disc. As described earlier, the disc is made up of two kinds of cartilage: a hard outer ring and a soft, spongy, liquidlike center. The discs give your back a buoyancy and the resilience to absorb between 500 and 1,500 pounds of shock, depending on your age. The bones and discs are held in place by thousands and thousands of ligament fibers that go from vertebra to vertebra. Each vertebra has two bony arms that meet in the back, enclosing a hole in the middle. These form a long canal, which houses and protects the spinal cord. Nerves, the messengers of our nervous system, exit from the spinal cord through an opening on the side of each vertebra.

There are about 2,000 muscles in the back and neck that control movement. Although pains in the back and neck are perceived as coming from the muscles, muscles in fact are rarely the cause of pain.

MUSCLE SPASM

The aching muscles in your back are rarely the main cause of back pain, even though they may feel rock hard. The

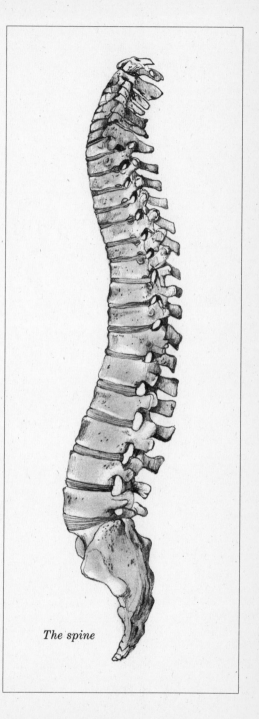

The spine

steellike knots that you feel are spastic muscles, which contract as an involuntary automatic response in the body to injury. This protective spasm is triggered when you make a movement that begins to impinge on the injured structure.

A muscle spasm doesn't help you to know what's injured. That's because a muscle spasm will occur with many kinds of injuries: a torn ligament or tendon, a disc pressing on a nerve, an irritation within a joint, an infection, or a severe tear in a muscle. When evaluating your injury, keep in mind that *a muscle spasm is a result of an injury, not an injury itself*. Actual tears of muscles in the back and neck area are fairly rare. Bone displacements, sprained and torn ligaments, poorly formed scar tissue, and ruptured discs pressing on nerves are the main causes of back and neck pains. Of course, diseases such as arthritis and cancer of the spine cause pain, but they occur less frequently.

REFERRED PAIN

You've probably forgotten what was on pages 6–8, about that odd phenomenon called referred pain and its connection with dermatomes—so now would be a good time to go back and reread it, because referred pain plays a large part in evaluating back and neck problems. When pain is referred in the body it takes a specific pathway, which is called a dermatome pattern. If you can trace the pathway of your pain and match it with one of the dermatome diagrams in this chapter, you will have a strong clue as to what you've injured.

An example of how pain travels can be seen in an injury to the base of the neck. If you have injured a nerve or ligament there, you may feel the pain in your neck but you may also feel it down the front or back of your arm. Perhaps you'll feel it *only* down your arm. This is because the back of the neck and the upper arm and forearm are part of the same dermatome—the C6 or C7 dermatome. An even stranger example is found when a disc in the lower part of the back presses on a nerve, or when a nearby

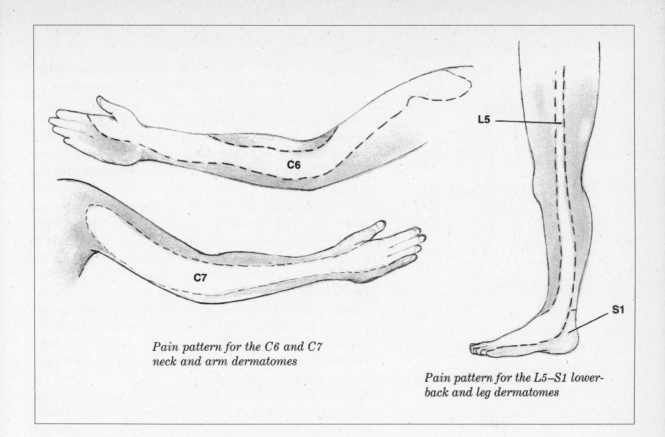

*Pain pattern for the C6 and C7
neck and arm dermatomes*

*Pain pattern for the L5–S1 lower-
back and leg dermatomes*

lower-back ligament is sprained. With either of these injuries you might feel pain down the outer part of your leg,
across your foot, and ending in your big toe. The connection between a pain in your toe and an injury in your lower
back can be difficult to imagine, but here again we are
dealing with a single—though twisted—dermatome pathway. How far the pain travels along a pathway is deter-
mined by how severe the injury is. You can feel pain in any
part of the dermatome. Also bear in mind that dermatomes are not exactly the same on everybody. They may
be in slightly different places in different people. Even
when you can follow the pathway of the dermatome back
to the injury, you may have difficulty determining if it's a
nerve or a ligament that you have injured, but there are

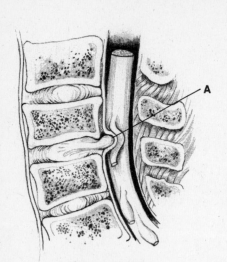

Disc protrusion

other indicators that will help you differentiate one injury from another once you've found the right dermatome.

THE SIGNIFICANCE OF WEAKNESS

When you feel like you've lost control of a part of your body because a muscle or group of muscles feel weak, it is usually a sign of serious trouble. One of your legs may feel as if it is going to collapse under you, or you might have trouble lifting things that you used to lift easily. Or you could get tired unusually fast doing something simple, such as trying to open a jar. This weakness can occur in an arm, hand, leg, or foot and is often accompanied by a noticeable change in the size of the muscle. When your muscle mass shrinks away it's called atrophy. Sometimes muscle atrophy and weakness is very obvious, but at times it is subtle and can hardly be noticed, especially in the beginning. When the root of the injury is in the back or neck, the weakness generally indicates that a ruptured (commonly called "slipped") disc (A) is pinching a nerve. The muscles receive their orders from the brain through the nervous system via electrical impulses. When a ruptured disc causes intense pressure on the nerve, the electrical impulses can no longer get through easily. The muscle cannot work properly, and a disintegration of muscle bulk and strength occurs.

One clear example of weakness in a lower-back injury is when control of the foot during walking is lost. This is commonly referred to as "foot drop"—the foot drags and flexing the foot is impossible.

If you feel weakness in a specific area it may also imply that your body is suffering from a serious disease. Whenever you feel weakness it is important to see a doctor as soon as possible.

PINS AND NEEDLES (TINGLING)

We all know that antsy feeling of pins and needles when your arm or leg falls asleep. This sensation, or tingling, can sometimes be a sign of serious trouble. When it indicates a serious problem, these sensations occur in your hands or your feet or both constantly. This often means that there is direct pressure on the spinal cord and you should see a doctor right away.

If the sensation of pins and needles is felt occasionally in one hand or foot or in your arm or leg, it is not necessarily serious. Most people have experienced this sensation after sitting in one position for too long. Your leg falls asleep as a result of pressure on the nerve in your thigh and the pins-and-needles sensation is only the waking up of the nerve once again.

STRUCTURAL ABNORMALITIES OF THE SPINE

SPONDYLOLISTHESIS

If you think this word is hard to say, you can imagine what it is like for some people to live with it. It's a congenital condition in which one of the vertebrae (A) is shoved substantially forward or back—either toward or away from the abdomen, instead of sitting squarely stacked on its neighbor. The vertebra may be one-quarter to one-half inch out of alignment, and although this distance may not sound so substantial, it can make for a lot of trouble. Imagine walking past a neatly stacked column of cans and pulling one of the central bottom cans slightly out of line. There may not be a sudden crash of cans, but there will be a lot of stress at the bottom of the column. The extra stress means that people with this condition are more vulnerable to injuries in this area. Usually this condition occurs in the lower back, but it can happen in the neck and midback, too.

KYPHOSIS

Kyphosis is an accentuated backward curve of the spine in the midback region—what literature and folk tradition calls a hunchback. Though the origin of this condition can

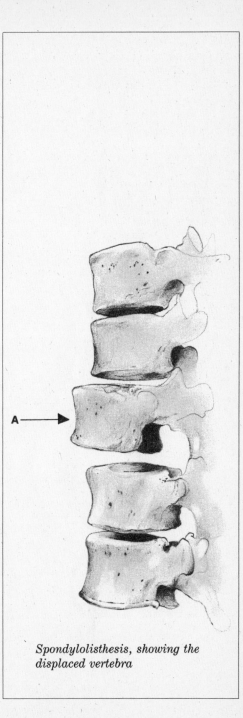

Spondylolisthesis, showing the displaced vertebra

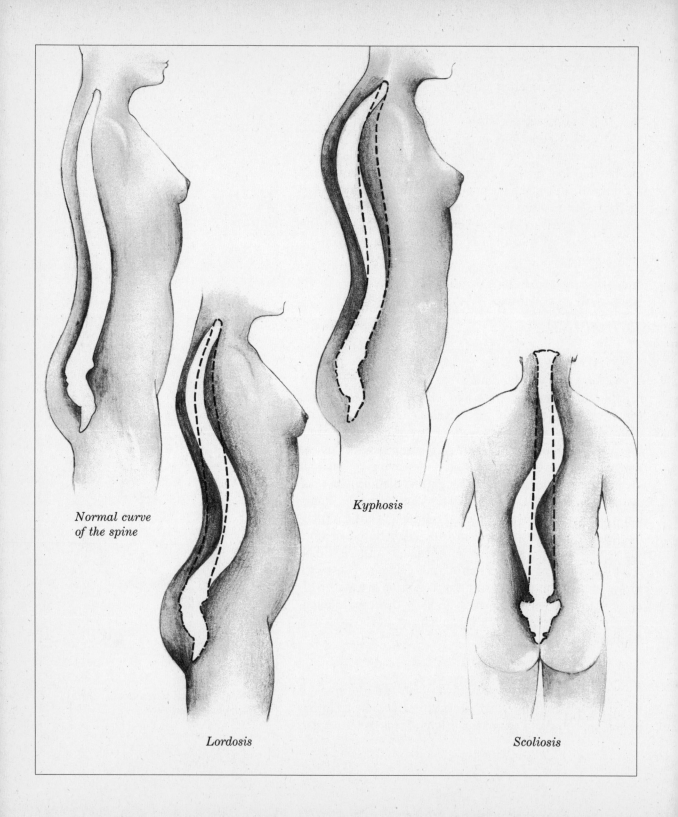

Normal curve
of the spine

Kyphosis

Lordosis

Scoliosis

be an inherited structural abnormality, in its milder form
it is more often the result of chronically poor posture and
lack of exercise. It would seem to follow that individuals
who have kyphosis would be more prone to injury in that
area, but in my experience, I have not seen any greater
incidence of injury among these cases.

LORDOSIS

The old gray mare with her swaying back and sagging posture is an exaggerated version of lordosis. Lordosis refers
to an exaggerated forward curve of the spine. Usually this
condition occurs in the lower back and is often called a
swayback. It is a postural problem rather than an inherited one. We all have a small forward curve of the lower
spine, which is normal and desirable; it's only when this
curve is accentuated that there may be problems. My experience leads me to believe that a chronic swayback can
lead to ligament injuries of the lower spine because the
backward projecting parts of the spine (spinous processes)
are jammed together in what is called "kissing spines."
This may place undue pressure on the ligaments and make
them more prone to injury, but this is just an educated
guess.

SCOLIOSIS

There is distortion and unnecessary worry about what scoliosis is and does. First of all, it is a sideways S curve of
the spine. This is often accompanied by a slight twisting of
the spine as well. When scoliosis is extreme, the muscles
of the back are developed unevenly with one side being
very muscular and the other side much less so. The body
develops in this way to make the spine as stable as possible. When scoliosis is slight this uneven development does
not happen. Extreme cases of scoliosis in children can be
very painful and often require surgery, but these cases are
infrequent. Millions of people have a very slight degree of
scoliosis curvature which *does not* affect the stability of
the spine or increase the likelihood of injury.

THE NECK

Neck pain is very confusing because it is often referred. In addition to a pain in your neck, a pain in your upper arm or hand can be caused by a neck injury. Even headaches and pain that is felt as far away as the inner side of the shoulder blade are also often caused by a problem in the neck. When discussing injuries to the neck, there will be diagrams of the dermatomes* so that you can match the pain pathways with your own.

People with pain in their arms, shoulders, head, hands, or midback often think they have injured themselves in those places. But many of them have injured their necks. The way to know if it's your neck that you've injured is to see if the pain comes on or gets worse when you move your head in certain directions, e.g. looking back over your shoulder, looking up at the ceiling, and so on. You may also have a neck injury if your neck hurts after you've been holding your head in certain positions for a long time; for example, typing, or holding a telephone between your shoulder and your ear. If, however, you feel pain when moving your arm to throw something, lift something, or take off clothing, your injury is most likely in your shoulder.

If this sounds as if it could get confusing, you're right. Neck and shoulder injuries are often confused with one another. Unfortunately, it's common to have both a neck and a shoulder injury at the same time, both creating a similar pain. To get rid of your pain it is important to discover both and treat them successfully—therefore you need to check for neck *and* shoulder injuries.

There are seven neck (cervical) vertebrae. If you put your fingers on one of the bony bumps on the lower part of your neck, you are touching the end of a long protruding bone, called the spinous process (A). There are similar extensions of bone going out on each side (B), but these you cannot feel readily with your hand. In addition, there are thousands of ligament fibers (C and D) that run between

*See p. 68.

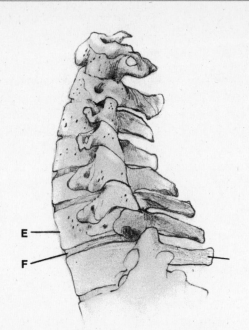

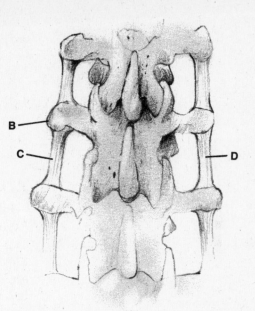

Neck vertebrae (side view), showing the spinous process (A), the body (E), and the disc (F)

Vertebrae and connecting ligaments—back view. . .

these extensions of bone and give the spine its strength and stability. See drawings above and on page 212.

Between the main bodies of the vertebrae (E) lie those famous shock-absorbing spongy discs (F). The discs in your neck are thicker than those in the midback. You need this extra cushioning because the neck is more vulnerable to injury and because it is capable of more varied movement. A disc has no feeling—when it is injured it doesn't cause pain. What happens is that the disc presses on a nerve, and *that* hurts. The nerves (G) exit through the small holes (H) between each of the vertebrae and keep branching out through the body. See next page.

There are muscles in the back of the neck that allow you to look up at the ceiling or kiss somebody taller than you are. There are those on the sides that help you turn your head, and more muscles in the front that help you bend your head forward. The muscles' primary function is to

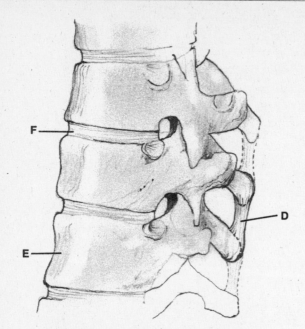

. . .and side view, showing the spinous process, the supraspinous ligament (D), the body of the vertebra (E), and the disc (F)

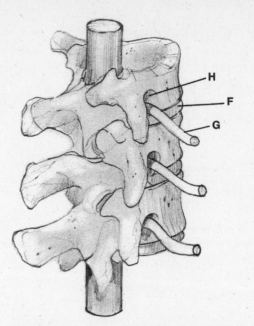

Spinal nerve exits, showing the disc (F), spinal nerve (G), and exit holes (H)

help you balance your head on top of your spine. The neck muscles aren't usually very strong because they don't have to be, except, of course, for wrestlers, boxers, and football players.

Although people often think neck pain comes from sore muscles in the neck, more often neck pain is caused by problems with discs, ligaments, nerves, and joints.

Ligament Injuries in the Neck

WHAT IS IT?

It's not only bad traffic jams or a houseful of screaming kids that gives you a pain in the neck. Microscopic tears of the ligaments of your neck are often the culprits. But because of the phenomenon of referred pain, you often feel the discomfort several inches away from the actual tearing. When you strain ligaments in your neck, the head and/or neck may ache on both sides, or the pain may be sharp on only one side. It can also radiate down toward the shoulder blade and even down the arm. You usually tear the ligaments at the back (A) and the sides (B) of the neck. Their function is to hold the vertebrae in your neck together, and they give the neck stability and strength.

HOW AND WHY

Severe neck injuries can hit you like a bolt of lightning and make you miserable for months. They can come as a result of a forceful accident, a head-on collision in an athletic event, a fall, or a car accident where whiplash may occur.

   (Whiplash is a generic term for an injury that occurs when

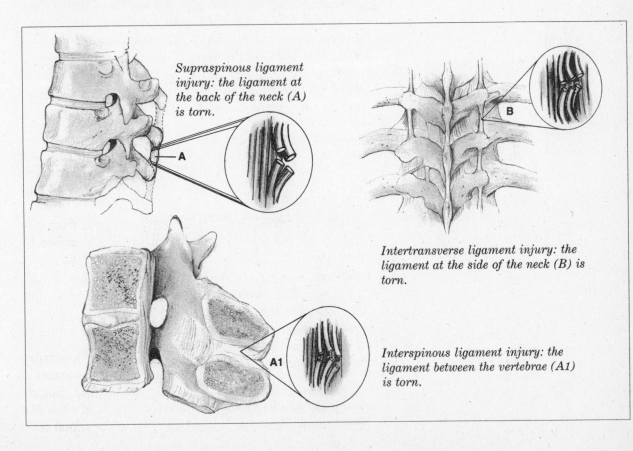

Supraspinous ligament injury: the ligament at the back of the neck (A) is torn.

Intertransverse ligament injury: the ligament at the side of the neck (B) is torn.

Interspinous ligament injury: the ligament between the vertebrae (A1) is torn.

the head is thrust violently forward and then snapped back.) All of these events cause tears in the ligaments, which can be quite painful.

Then there's the kind of neck pain that comes on slowly, for no apparent reason. Frequently the ligaments are weakened over a period of months or years if they are forcefully stretched beyond their limit, as they are in shoulder stands, plow positions, and so on. They are also weakened if a person is chronically tense and holds that tension in his neck. The tension hampers circulation, and this affects the mobility and general health of the neck.* Frequently people wake up with a neck pain from sleeping in an awkward position that has unnaturally stretched their ligaments. The body tries to protect the torn ligaments by having the muscles in the area involuntarily go into spasm. The spasm limits your movement, which protects you from further damage. This often accounts for the feeling of stiffness in the neck. At times it's difficult to differentiate neck pain caused by ligament tears from pain caused by disc problems, because they both give rise to similar pain symptoms.

DIAGNOSTIC VERIFICATION

When you test your neck you are looking for two things: first, what movements cause you pain? and second, is your movement restricted in one or more directions? This will often differentiate a ligament tear from a disc problem. Do all of the following tests standing up.

Test 1

First, look as far to the right and the left as you can. Look up to the ceiling, down to the floor. Tilt your head to the right, then the left, trying to bring your ear toward your shoulder (don't cheat by raising your shoulder to your ear). These tests are designed to give you a general idea of the movements that cause you discomfort.

---

*The Neck Relaxer is a device that is very effective in reducing neck tension and pain. Available from Relaxation Tools, Inc., P.O. Box 1045, New York, N.Y. 10025.

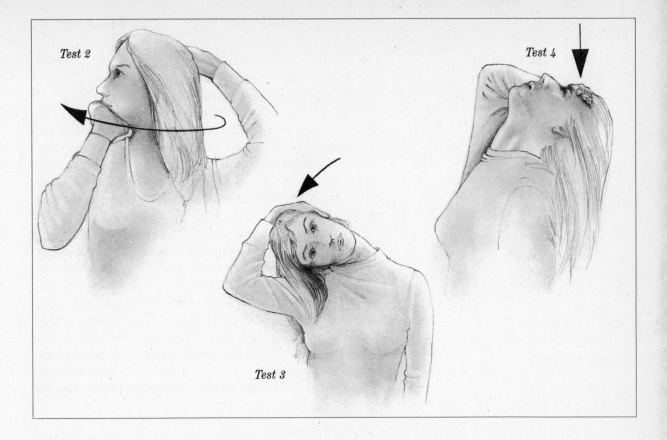

Test 2
Now place one hand behind your head, and the other one on your chin, as in the drawing, and turn your head to one side as fully as possible. Do not use your neck muscles. Let your hands do the work. Repeat to the other side. There is usually more pain in one direction than in another.

Test 3
Now tilt your head to the right side and place your right hand on the side of your head above your right ear and press down gently. Repeat to the other side. Note the differences.

Test 4
Now look up to the ceiling and place one hand on your forehead. Push back and down gently so that your face is flat to the ceiling. Stop if you feel pain.

Test 5

Now drop your head slowly toward your chest. Place one hand on the back of your head and push down very gently. Never push so hard as to give yourself severe pain.

A healthy neck has full range of motion in all directions. It should be able to turn 180° from side to side. You should also be able to have your ear almost touch your shoulder, and when looking up you should have the range shown in the drawing. With advancing age this range becomes slightly decreased.

If you can move your neck with your hand fairly fully in all directions, even though this will cause pain, it is most likely that you have a ligament tear. If, however, there is a severe restriction in movement in one direction but not in the opposite direction, it's fairly likely you have a disc problem, especially if you have pain down the arm as well.

To be candid, you may find it tough to differentiate one from the other. However, the pain patterns illustrated on these pages may help you find which ligament is injured if the path of your pain corresponds to any one of the patterns.

Medical Treatment

There is no effective self-treatment that I know.

1. DEEP FRICTIONING AND DEEP MASSAGE: Frictioning of the superficial ligaments is often effective. Deep massage of the muscles is very helpful when tension is an important factor.
2. INJECTION: A series of three to six proliferant injections into the ligaments of the neck is a very effective treatment. Over six or eight weeks the proliferant thickens and strengthens the ligaments.*
3. TRACTION: Intermittent traction is often effective as a temporary solution.
4. MANIPULATION: If it is not effective within three to five treatments it is probably not going to work for you.

---

*Unfortunately only very few physicians are skilled at neck injections of this type.

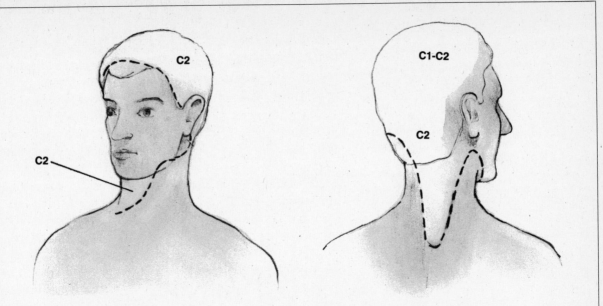

Neck-injury pain pattern: if you feel pain in this area (the C1 and C2 cervical dermatomes), you may have injured the ligament that attaches the first or second cervical vertebra.

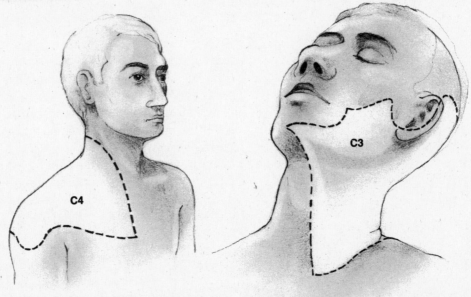

Neck-injury pain patterns: if it hurts here, you have probably injured the ligaments of the third (C3) or fourth (C4) vertebra.

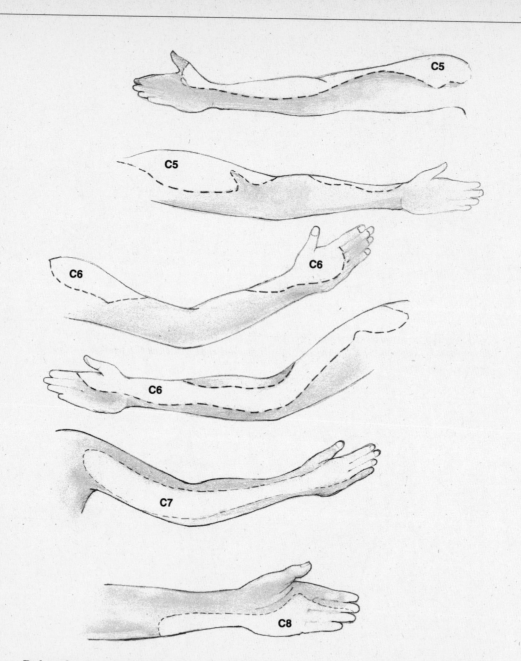

Referred-pain patterns from neck-ligament injuries. The numbers refer to the probable ligament area of your injury—the fifth, sixth, or seventh cervical vertebra. These pain-reference patterns are often present in addition to pain felt in the neck. They can also be present without pain felt in the neck.

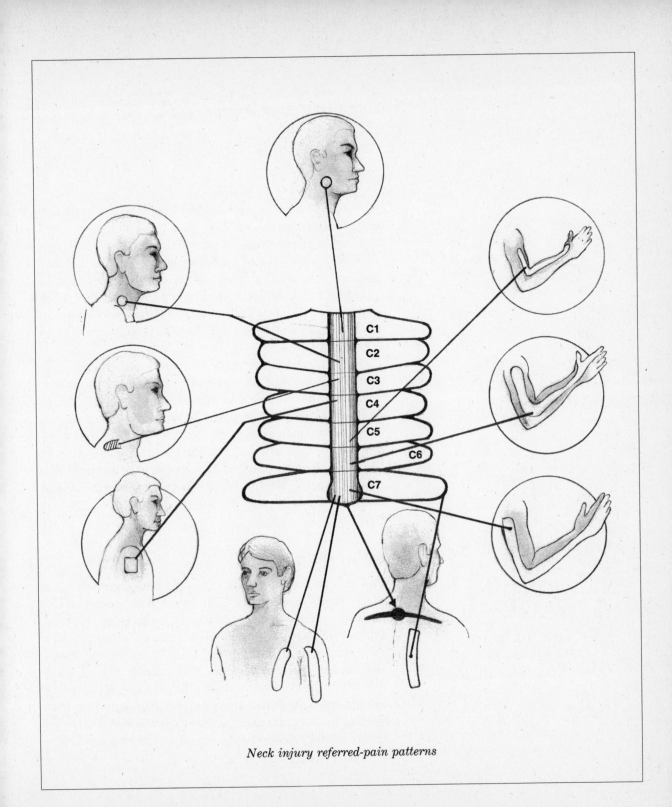

Neck injury referred-pain patterns

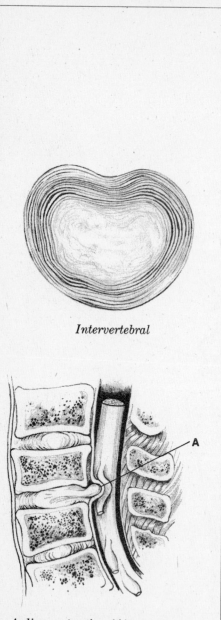

Intervertebral

A disc protrusion (A) can press on a nerve and cause pain.

Disc Injuries in the Neck
(Pinched Nerve)

WHAT IS IT?

When I was a teenager I was in a small dance company. Once I was performing a waltz with this group, and before the show I was seized with a stiff, painful neck. Since I couldn't turn my head without turning my body, I was hardly a graceful figure and stood out like a sore thumb. To make it look as though this was part of the dance, the director had us dance as if we all had stiff necks. It's one of the rare instances where a likely disc problem was put to creative use.

Discs are shock-absorbing soft cartilages (see illustration) that separate each of the vertebrae of the spine. When a disc is injured (A) it cracks and a piece of it protrudes. If this piece compresses a nearby nerve, it can cause severe pain in the neck, or refer the pain to the upper back or arm. Although there are six different discs in the neck, the ones near the base of the neck are most frequently injured, for this is the seat of most movement and stress.

HOW AND WHY

One woman I worked with said, "My neck pain on a scale of one to ten is an eleven." However, disc injuries in the neck are unpredictable. Your pain could be a two or a three, could last for years or bother you for about ten days each month. The whole ordeal could start from a night's sleep in an awkward position. You wake to find you have difficulty turning your head without pain. Other beginning signals are pain that starts after reading or typing with the head in a bent position. These are the slow-emerging disc problems. No one really knows why they occur. Other neck injuries occur through accidents, such as a fall or whiplash injury.*

If the disc is strongly pressing on the nerve, the pain may be felt radiating all the way down the arm. You may have a feeling of "pins and needles" in your hand or fingers and have a weakness in some of the muscles of the arm or hand that are controlled by the nerve being pinched.

Except in the case of accidents, we don't really know what causes disc injuries. But the most convincing theory I know of results from a study done by Frank Pierce Jones† that clearly shows that people with compressed, sagging postures have increased pressure on their discs. Since the central part of the disc is fairly flexible and liquidlike, constant pressure would make the disc want to bulge out in all directions. This in turn weakens the structure of the ligaments that surround the disc, and the whole area becomes more vulnerable to injury.

DIAGNOSTIC VERIFICATION

In many cases it is very difficult to distinguish between disc and ligament injuries in the neck. One common indicator of a disc injury is that you can turn your head in one direction fairly easily but you can't turn it in the opposite direction because the pain is so severe. With ligament injuries there may be difficulty turning the head, but you can do it. Another fairly certain indicator of disc injuries is a weakening of the muscles of the arm or hand. In spite of these indicators it may be tough to know whether you've

---

*Whiplash only describes the way in which the injury occurs. It describes a type of motion rather than a specific injury. This motion is a sudden forward-and-back snapping of the neck, which occurs most frequently from a rear-end collision. Whiplash can cause injuries to the discs or ligaments, or both.

†*Body Awareness in Action: A Study of the Alexander Technique* (New York, 1976).

injured a disc or ligament in your neck, and it is advised that you consult a physician.

Tests

This weakness could be very obvious, or it could be so subtle that even a physician would have a difficult time. See page 214, because the tests are identical to those used for ligaments. There are other tests that differentiate between ligament and disc injuries in the neck, but they are too difficult and involved to do yourself.

The pain patterns illustrated below can help you find which disc is injured if the path of your pain corresponds to one of the patterns. Patterns of pain felt in the arm usually accompany a pain in the neck.

TREATMENT CHOICES

Self-Treatment

Unfortunately, the treatment choices for disc injuries are extremely limited. There are a few things you can do to minimize your pain. One is to avoid positions that cause you pain. Do not read or write or type with your head bent forward if this has been troubling you. Instead, keep your head erect by reading with a book held close to eye level or writing on a tilted surface (a miniature drafting table works well) or an inexpensive lap desk.* When typing, always use a music stand placed directly behind the typewriter at eye level, or use a special clipboard attachment, sold in good stationery stores, called a copy-holder. This will ensure that your head is never twisted and bent forward. Always sleep with a pillow that keeps your head in line with your spine. You need a thicker pillow if you sleep on your side than if you sleep on your back. It's best not to sleep on your stomach, because to do this you have to twist your head.

---

*Lap desks can be obtained from Relaxation Tools, Inc., P.O. Box 1045, New York, N.Y. 10025.

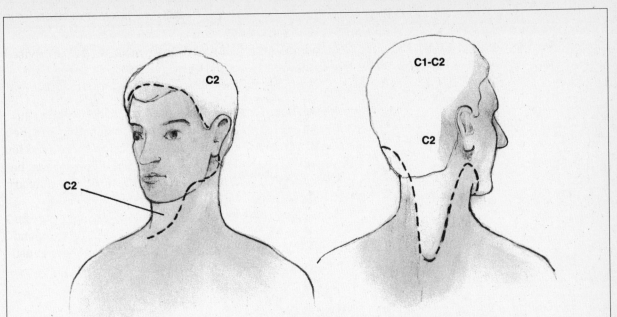

Pain in these areas means that your disc injury is probably located at the first or second cervical disc.

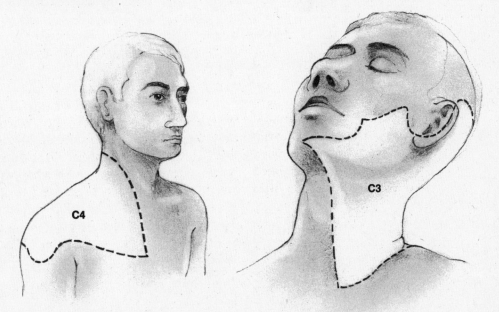

Pain in these areas probably means an injury at the third or fourth cervical disc.

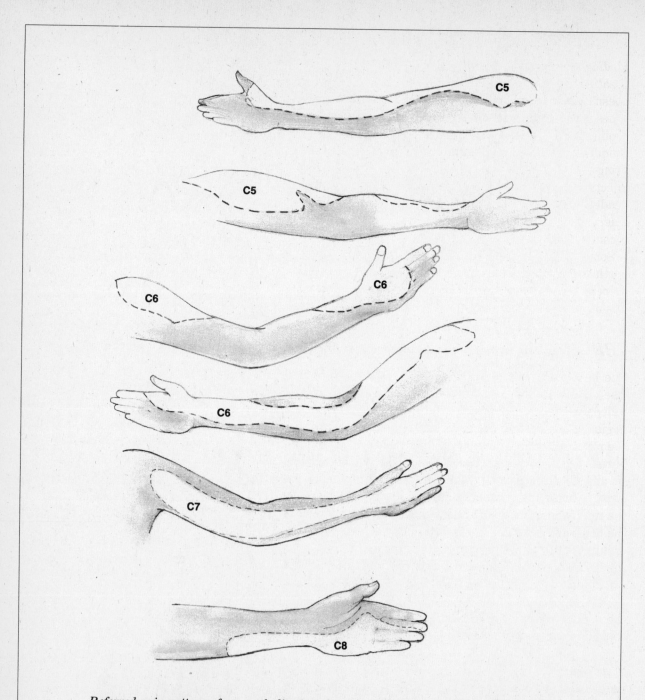

Referred-pain patterns from neck-disc injuries. You may feel pain in these areas in addition to—or instead of—pain in your neck if you've injured a disc.

Medical Treatment

Treating disc injuries in the neck is very rough. There just doesn't seem to be any definitive way to treat them. At times manipulation seems to bring relief. In some cases proliferant injections to strengthen the ligaments surrounding the disc are helpful. Neck traction can either bring relief or make you worse. When pain is severe, an injection can be given into the nerve, which completely deadens the nerve being pinched by the disc. This is called a nerve block. In some cases surgery to remove the disc is recommended.

Sometimes time takes care of it, because the protruding portion of the disc dries up and is reabsorbed by the body, thereby releasing the pressure on the nerve. However, this often takes up to a year.

THE MIDBACK

The hunchback of Notre Dame had a midback problem. The overaccentuated curve that marks the hunchback is called kyphosis. The portion of the back called the midback begins at the base of the neck and goes to the bottom of the rib cage, where it meets the lower back. It has twelve vertebrae (A) with a rib attached to either side of each one (B and C). This part of your back can barely bend and twist because the vertebrae are solidly fixed in place by the ribs, which is a good arrangement because it protects the lungs and heart.

Injuries in the midback are less common than those in the neck and low back because of this limited mobility. A great deal of pain in the midback area, also called the thoracic area, can be caused by referred pain from injuries to the neck. For instance, pain between the shoulder blades could be the result of a whiplash injury to the neck.

Many pains that occur in this area are due to disease or disturbances of the internal organs (such as heart attack, lung cancer, pneumonia, etc.), so it is especially important to see your doctor if you suffer pain in the midback, even if

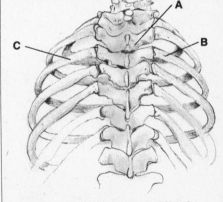

The thoracic spine, or midback region, showing the thoracic vertebrae (A) and the ribs (B and C)

you think it's from an athletic injury. For instance, muscle injuries in this area often create pain when you breathe deeply—but so does pneumonia.

Ligament Injuries to the Midback

WHAT IS IT?

The occupational hazard of secretaries and typists is often the desk disease of an aching midback. When you have a pain across the middle of your back it can be from strain and tearing of the ligaments that attach your vertebrae to one another. Even though the strain is in the area of the spine, pain may be referred outwards in one or both directions, creating a generalized aching feeling, or a sharp pain that can even travel around toward the chest.

HOW AND WHY

How many people do you know who sit or stand with a sagging back and collapsed chest? Probably quite a few. This posture often causes a slow stretching and loss of healthy tone in the ligaments. Because the ligaments have been weakened, they won't handle stress very well. When they are suddenly called upon to do some work, they may strain easily. Pain that originates in this way usually feels like a dull ache. It frequently comes on after sitting or working over a desk for thirty minutes to an hour.

Accidents and fatigue injuries in this area are not uncommon, especially for people who do heavy work such as construction. Also, I've often seen it happen in those who practice tennis serves by the hour. Any fall that violently twists the upper body can cause a slight tear or strain of the ligaments. Midback ligament injuries most commonly occur when you're bent over in an awkward position lifting something heavy, and twist to put it somewhere else. A sharp, searing pain occurs when the ligament is suddenly torn.

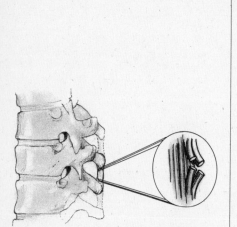

Injury to the supraspinous ligament

DIAGNOSTIC VERIFICATION

Test
Straddle a chair facing the back and hold onto the back of the chair while you twist your upper body around and look behind you. Use your arms and not your back muscles to do the twisting. Do this forcefully in both directions. This is usually the most painful test in midback ligament injuries. Because of the many internal organs and complications of referred pain from the neck, a physician should check you out when you have pain in this area. If you have injured a ligament, you may have one of the pain patterns illustrated on pages 228, 230, and 231.

TREATMENT CHOICES

Self-Treatment
If you've had an accident followed by a sharp pain, you may choose to rest for several weeks until it goes away. If it doesn't disappear by itself within a reasonable length of time, rest will not be effective.

Medical Treatment
1. MANIPULATION: In some cases, one or two manipulations seem to eradicate the pain. Why this is so, I cannot say. But I've seen it work in many instances.
2. INJECTION: Injections of proliferant into the strained ligaments are very effective. But it usually takes three or four treatments before you feel relief.

Rehabilitation
Do all back exercises daily when you can do them without pain (pp. 272–76).

Disc Injuries to the Midback

WHAT IS IT?

Sudden, severe midback injuries can feel like a heart attack, creating a knifelike pain through the chest. When a

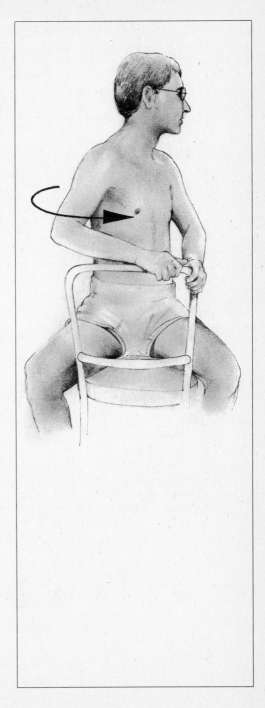

Midback referred-pain patterns: if you feel pain in any of these areas, you may have strained one of your midback ligaments.

disc in the midback area is damaged and part of it presses
on a nerve coming out from the spine, pain, numbness,
and/or burning sensations can result. Depending on which
disc is injured in the midback, pain and discomfort can be
felt in varying places—one side of the midback, straight
across the midback, between the shoulder blades, through
the midback to the chest, or just below the shoulder blade
traveling around the midback to the chest.

Fortunately, because of the limited movement in this
area, discs in the midback are damaged much less frequently than those in the neck and lower back. When
there is pain in this region it is usually due to injury to the
ligaments.

HOW AND WHY

As with so many other problems, no one really knows why
injuries occur in the midback region. One possible cause is
a constant slouched posture, especially in those who sit at
a desk all day, year after year. This poor posture weakens
the surrounding ligaments that hold the disc in place, making a disc protrusion more likely. Of course, a severe auto-
mobile accident can cause a midback disc to rupture, but
this is fairly rare. One case in which the cause of the disc
problem was obvious was that of a young man who had
been shoveling a heavy load, ten hours a day. After six
weeks of this, his disc ruptured and he felt a searing pain
starting in his midback and traveling out to his side with
an accompanying numbness.

DIAGNOSTIC VERIFICATION

Differentiating a disc injury from a ligament strain in this
area has its problems. Both produce a similar pain that is
exacerbated by twisting or by a deep breath or cough, but
the disc injury will usually produce numbness, or a pain
that wraps around the chest, and/or arm pain. Follow the
same testing procedure as for ligament injuries (p. 227);
unfortunately, all this will tell you is whether your injury
is in your midback rather than referred from the neck. The

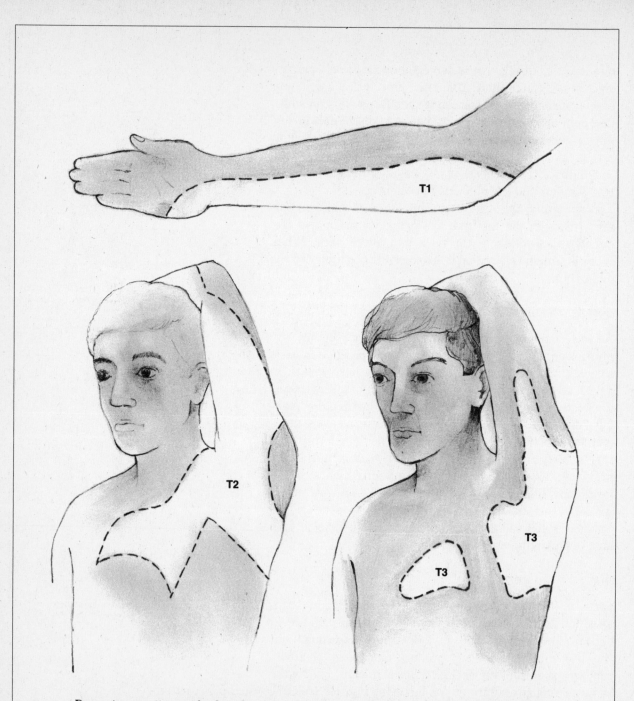

Dermatome patterns of referred pain: pain in any of these areas means probable injury at the first (T1), second (T2), or third (T3) ligament or disc.

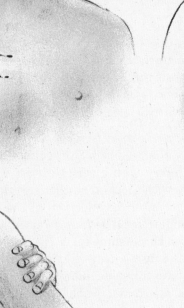

Common midback referred-pain patterns: pain here means probable injury at the tenth (T10) or eleventh (T11) thoracic vertebra

Common midback referred-pain patterns: pain here means probable injury at the fifth (T5) or fourth (T4) thoracic vertebra.

good news is that less than 2 percent of all midback injuries are disc problems. As mentioned before, it's important to consult a doctor when you have midback pain to rule out disease.

TREATMENT CHOICES

Self-Treatment

Often disc injuries are self-healing within one year. The disc material that has pushed out of its casing dries up and is reabsorbed by the body. Waiting for this to happen may be a boring and depressing prospect, but many believe there is little else you can do for yourself with this injury.

Medical Treatment

A physician can help differentiate between a ligament and disc injury with a series of test injections into the ligaments with a local anaesthetic. If the pain temporarily disappears after an injection, all, or at least part, of your discomfort could be from strained ligaments, which can be treated successfully (p. 227).

If the disc is only slightly dislodged, proliferant injections into the surrounding ligaments can sometimes tighten the ligaments, pushing the disc off the nerve.

Muscle Injuries to the Midback

WHAT IS IT?

"I pulled a muscle in my back. These weekends in the yard are killing me." Though the complaint is common, pulled muscles in the midback are not usually the source of your pain. However, when muscle injuries do occur in the midback area, they are usually due to a strain of one of the muscles in between the ribs (A) and occasionally muscles of the shoulder blade, which attach to the spine (B). In the case of rib-muscle strain, the pain is sharp and is usually on one side of the back near the bottom of the shoulder blade. It is sometimes felt piercing straight through the

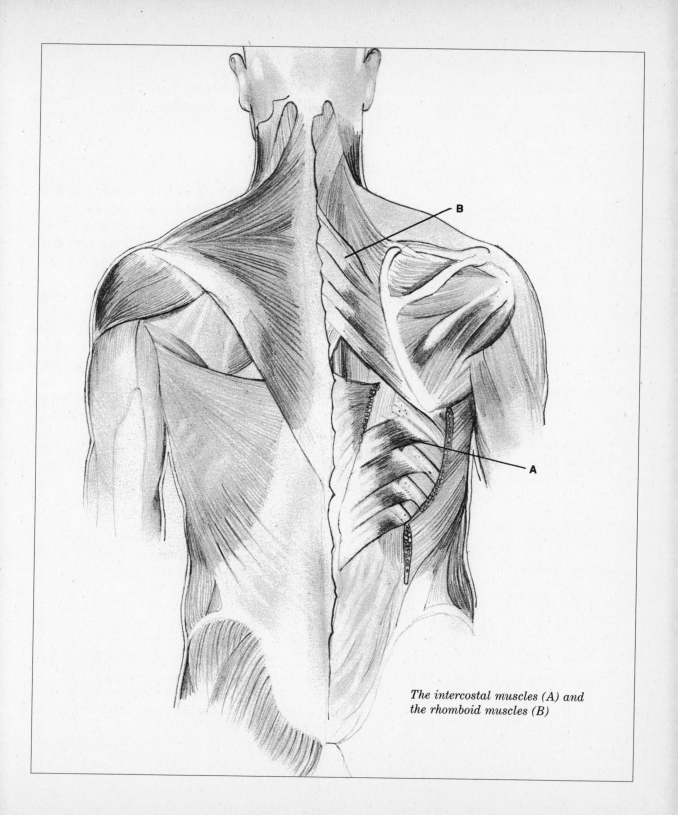

*The intercostal muscles (A) and
the rhomboid muscles (B)*

chest. These small muscles between the ribs, called intercostal muscles, help us breathe and help stabilize the chest when lifting things.

HOW AND WHY

A piercing pain in the midback region is usually felt after unusually vigorous athletic activity, a sudden twist, or exertion in an awkward position. It also happens when lifting something heavy, especially if you almost drop it and catch it again. With this injury, inhaling deeply often causes a sharp pain.

The aching discomfort felt between the shoulder blades, if it's muscular in origin, is from the strain that occurs over a fairly long period of time. This type of discomfort is often difficult to differentiate from ligament strain, for the pain or discomfort from both is similar. Pain in the shoulder-blade area can also be a referred pain from injuries to the neck, as discussed in the previous section. Another possible reason for general discomfort across the upper part of the midback is an accumulation of excess muscle tension, often caused by poor posture and emotional stress. All these factors make it somewhat difficult for you to evaluate pain in this region without help.

DIAGNOSTIC VERIFICATION

Because of the complexity of evaluating this injury, as described above, a doctor's help should be sought.

TREATMENT CHOICES

Self-Treatment

In the case of intercostal strain, rest from activities that cause pain and the avoidance of very deep breathing for one to two weeks is usually all that's needed. In cases of strain in the muscles between the shoulder blades, rest is usually ineffective.

Medical Treatment

1. DEEP MASSAGE AND DEEP FRICTIONING: Various massage techniques applied directly to the strained area usually help it heal more quickly. It is especially helpful in the case of rib-muscle strain.

2. INJECTION: When a build-up of poor scar tissue does not permit the pain to resolve itself, one, or at the most two, injections of either corticosteroids or proliferant are usually very effective.

THE LOWER BACK

The Mystery of Lower-Back Pain

It remains a mystery why lower-back pain occurs. We have clues but no answers. Some feel that it is strictly a mechanical phenomenon, i.e., just fatigue and strain of muscles and ligaments. Some feel it is caused by emotional stress. Still others think that a ruptured or slipped disc is the troublemaker. But no one understands *why* these things occur. Many different kinds of treatment, from exercise to surgery, claim success, but the plain truth is that most people who experience back pain have had some kind of pain in their backs off and on for years and years, despite the type of treatment they receive. There is no doubt that some forms of treatment are more effective than others in particular cases, but even here we don't know why. For example, it is clear that some people are helped by daily exercise regimes, while others aren't. In many cases injections seem to work wonders, but in similar cases they may not work at all.

It has been documented that emotional stress can precipitate an attack of back pain, but here again the reasons are cloudy. We are just beginning to understand the role of the psyche and the emotions in pain. One theory that explains how the emotions can directly affect pain is based on the fact that our adrenal glands produce the hormone cortisone, which constantly acts to "de-inflame" tissues that become irritated in the body. When we are under emotional stress the adrenal glands' cortisone function becomes disrupted, causing a decrease in this cortisone production. According to this theory, the decreased cortisone activity is the major factor in recurrent pains of many types.

Lower-Back Structure*

You might say my career started when I injured my back at thirteen. It took me twenty years, astounding as that sounds, to find someone who knew what was wrong with it. The lower-back area—also called the lumbar region—is the source of more pain than any other place in the body. The lumbar region (C) begins just beneath the back of the rib cage and ends at the top of the hip bones, where the sacrum (A) begins. I used to think my lower back ended somewhere in the middle of my hips and it wasn't until I began to study anatomy that I discovered that the lower back is only about six inches long in an average-sized adult. There are five vertebrae (C) in the lower back. These are abbreviated L1, L2, L3, L4, and L5 as an easy shorthand.

Together the five lower-back vertebrae form a forward curve, so that when you lie flat on your back on the floor with your legs straight you can easily slide your hand under your lower back. This curve is natural and necessary for the health of the lower back. I can remember feeling deformed in my gym classes in school because my lower back didn't touch the floor. Recent research in the functioning of the spine has shown that flattening your lower back lessens the balance and stability of the spine. It can actually make you prone to back pain by altering the natural position of the spine.

*Before reading this section, be sure to review the introduction to the spine, pp. 202ff., and the section on referred pain and dermatomes, pp. 6–8.

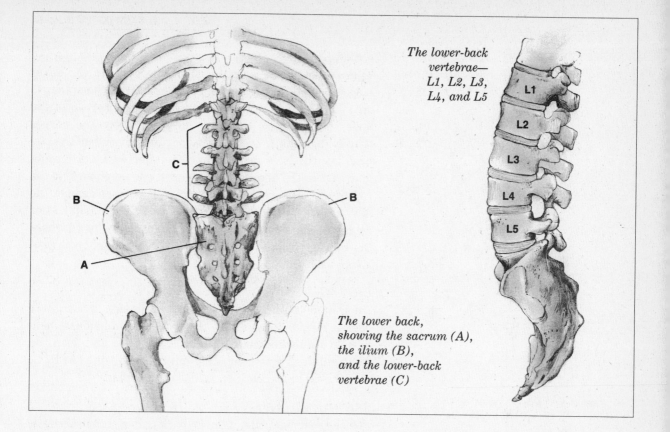

The lower-back
vertebrae—
L1, L2, L3,
L4, and L5

L1
L2
L3
L4
L5

The lower back,
showing the sacrum (A),
the ilium (B),
and the lower-back
vertebrae (C)

DISCS

A "slipped disc" is a popular misnomer. Discs almost never slip, though they crack and ooze and cause pressure on nerves. The discs that lie between the lower-back verte-brae are like half-dollar-sized plastic bags filled with a squishy substance that looks like crab meat. They hydrau-lically cushion the movement of all the bones. These lum-bar discs are the thickest of all the spinal discs, because they absorb the most weight. They conform to the shape of the natural forward curve, and are thicker in front to-ward your belly than they are in the back. This is a good arrangement: it keeps the pressure of the discs away from the nerves that exit from the spine toward the back of the vertebrae.

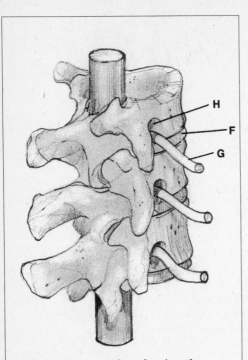

Spinal nerve exits, showing the disc (F), the spinal nerve (G), and the nerve exits (H)

NERVES

There's not much room for the nerves (G) in the lower back to come through their openings (H) in the spine, so any pinching of their space is crucial. The nerves of the lower back control the hips, legs, and feet. The nerves that exit beneath the fourth and fifth lower-back vertebrae are the ones most frequently affected by disc problems. Discs (F) and nerves (G) are close neighbors. If the rim of the disc cracks and a part of it presses against the nerve, either back, hip, leg, or foot pain, or numbness or weakness can result. Another ligament (D), which anchors the L5 vertebra to the pelvic bones, is a frequent source of lower-back pain.

LIGAMENTS

Another potential source of aches and pains in the lower back is strained ligaments. Several sets of ligaments help to hold the lower-back vertebrae together and keep the spine stable. Three commonly injured ligaments (A, B, C) are located at the back and sides of the spine.

SACRAL LIGAMENTS

But the main culprits of lower-back pain are the sacroiliac ligaments. These are the ones I searched twenty years to find. The sacrum (A), a triangular-shaped bone at the base of the spine, is wedged in between the hip or iliac bones (B). Sacroiliac ligaments (C) get their name by attaching the sacrum to the iliac (hip) bones. This crisscrossing mass of ligaments can be strained in many ways in dozens of places.

MUSCLES

The sets of muscles we are about to discuss are tongue twisters: the erector, the quadratus, and the iliopsoas. There are three sets of muscles that control movement in the lower back and pelvis. The erector spinae (A) is a group of muscles that run vertically on either side of the spine, and consist of hundreds of small muscles that go from vertebra to vertebra. The quadratus lumborum (B) attaches the top of the pelvis to several lower-back verte-

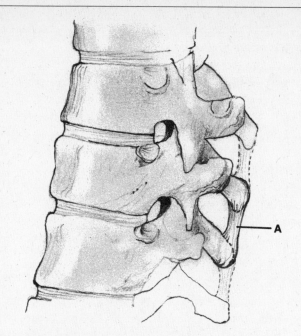

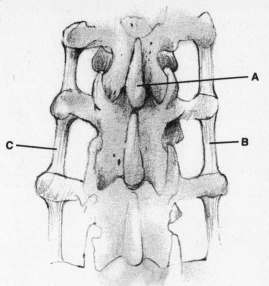

Supraspinous ligament (A) side view

Supraspinous ligament (A) back view and intertransverse ligaments (B and C)

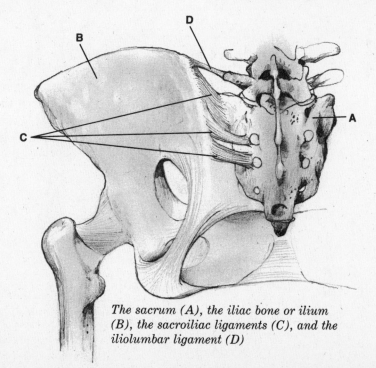

The sacrum (A), the iliac bone or ilium (B), the sacroiliac ligaments (C), and the iliolumbar ligament (D)

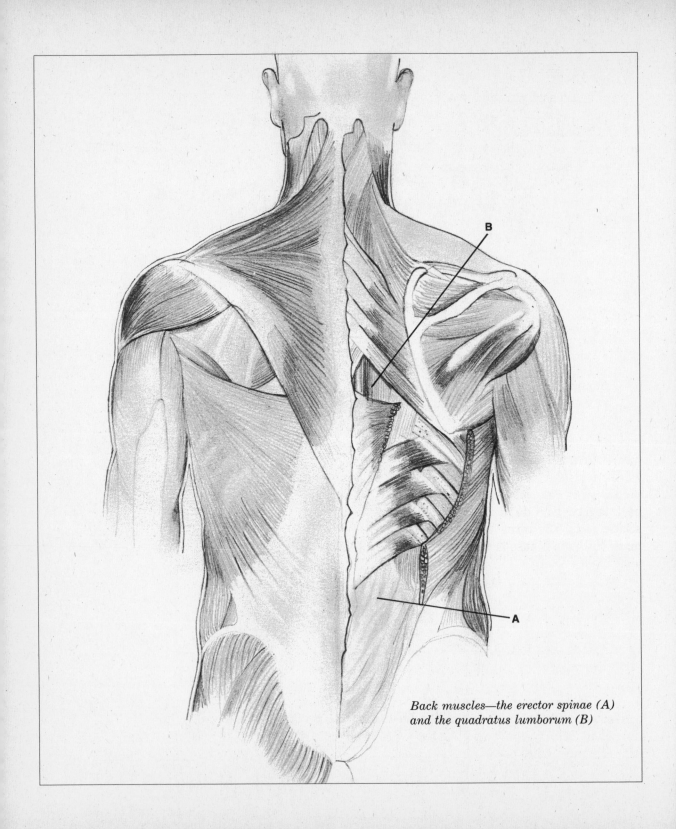

Back muscles—the erector spinae (A) and the quadratus lumborum (B)

brae. The iliopsoas group runs from several lower-back vertebrae through the pelvis to the inside of the thigh bone. These muscles can become strained and irritated and cause pain, but this is very rare. These are the muscles that frequently go into spasm when a disc or ligament is damaged. This spasm, or involuntary contraction, is a protective mechanism that tries to prevent movement that might increase the pain.

Lower-Back Ligament Tears

WHAT IS IT?

The plaguing pain in your back more often than not is caused by tears in the ligaments. As discussed in the introductory section, the lower-back region is composed of five lumbar vertebrae and the sacrum. Although the majority of lower-back pain actually originates in the sacral ligaments (A), tears to low-back ligaments (E) at L1 through L5 can be very painful. This lower-back pain may be accompanied by pain felt either in the buttock, thigh, lower leg, foot, or a combination of these areas. But these areas can be painful even when your back doesn't hurt and the pain is still being caused by ligament tears in the lower-back region. Pain down the leg is often called sciatica or sciatic pain. The term "sciatica" is not a diagnosis, for many things can cause it. It merely means a pain down the leg.

The ligaments most frequently torn are those between L4 and L5, or L5 and S1 (B and C), which run between the vertebrae, or the ligament (D) that holds the L5 vertebra to the side of the pelvis. Depending on the location of the tears, you may experience pain on either one or both sides of the lower back. Whether your pain radiates into the hip, thigh, and/or lower leg depends on which ligament is strained and on how badly it's injured. If a ligament is injured on one side only, you will feel pain on that side; if it is injured in the center or on both sides of the spine, pain is felt across the entire back or on the spine.

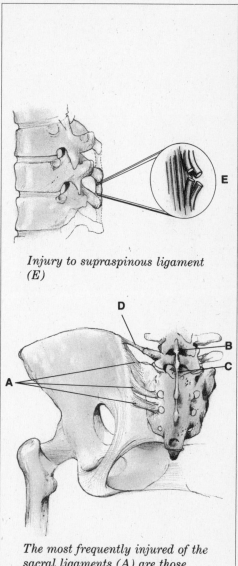

Injury to supraspinous ligament (E)

The most frequently injured of the sacral ligaments (A) are those between the fourth and fifth lumbar vertebra (B) or between the fifth lumbar and first sacral vertebra (C), or the iliolumbar ligament (D).

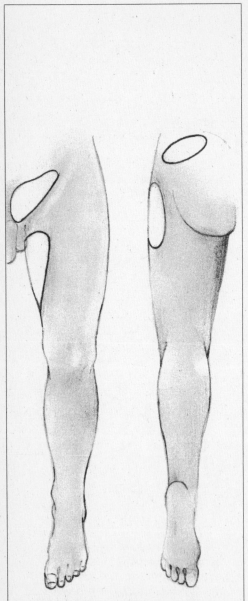

Referred-pain pattern for injury to the iliolumbar ligament (see previous illustration)

HOW AND WHY

Many of the same activities can cause different kinds of back problems. If you suffer from a fall or suddenly lift a heavy object, you may feel pain in the back immediately. If you're in the heat of a sports activity and sprain your ligament, you may not feel anything at all until many hours later, and then you won't be sure of how you hurt yourself. When the area is warmed up, ligament pain is often not perceptible. This is a phenomenon that many dancers and athletes will attest to.

Lower-back pain may persist or come and go with different kinds of activity. Often, prolonged sitting causes the lower back to ache, and lifting a heavy object may start a new bout of back pain.

Physiologically, a ligament will tear if it becomes fatigued or if more work is demanded of the ligament than it is capable of doing. A physical precondition for injury can be created by poor alignment, excess muscle tension, poor exercise habits, or weakness. When back pain recurs many times, it is frequently because the ligaments have healed with poorly formed scar tissue which is brittle and easily tears again and again under stress.

DIAGNOSTIC VERIFICATION

When ligament D is torn, pain can radiate to the groin, testicle, and inner thigh as well as into one side of the lower back, hip, and outer thigh. By yourself, you'll find it is difficult, if not impossible, to tell exactly which ligament is torn or to rule out a disc problem. This takes a physician who is knowledgeable and experienced in this field. What you can tell by yourself is if you've hurt a ligament. To determine this, bend forward and back and to each side, stopping as soon as you feel pain. With ligament tears, you'll probably feel pain in one or two directions.

When one of the lower-back ligaments is injured, the pain is usually in the lower back or hip or directly on the spine. Occasionally it can be referred down the leg. With

ligament strains to the lower back there are no pins or
needles or weakness in the legs or feet. But unless the
weakness is advanced it's hard to discern. The pain patterns illustrated on p. 242 may help you find which ligament is injured if the path of your pain corresponds to one
of these patterns.

TREATMENT CHOICES

Self-Treatment
Time, the healer of many wounds, may take care of this
injury temporarily. Unfortunately, it frequently returns
because of poor scar-tissue formation. Most people stop
any activity that causes them pain, which is a good idea.
For a real resolution to this problem you need professional
help.

Medical Treatment
1. MANIPULATION: Manipulation often helps ligament
   strains. One theory for why it works is that it re-
   aligns the bones and reduces undue stress on the ligaments. Another is that it tears improperly formed
   scar tissue, giving it a chance to heal more strongly.
2. DEEP MASSAGE: Deep massage on the lower-back region often helps to reduce or eliminate pain. Again
   we don't know why there is relief, but it's likely that
   the increased circulation speeds the ligaments' healing process when the strained ligament is near the
   surface.
3. INJECTION: Proliferant injections are very effective in
   eliminating the pain from strained ligaments. It usually takes from three to six injections over a period of
   one to two months for this treatment to work fully.
   Proliferants make the ligaments stronger and help
   prevent the recurrence of strain.

Rehabilitation
If not painful, do Back Series 1. When you are well, do all
back exercises daily (pp. 272–76).

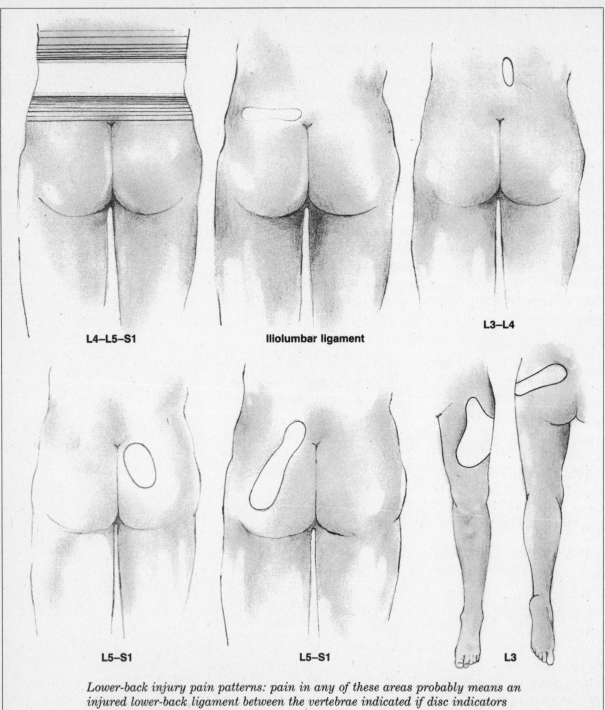

L4–L5–S1

Iliolumbar ligament

L3–L4

L5–S1

L5–S1

L3

Lower-back injury pain patterns: pain in any of these areas probably means an injured lower-back ligament between the vertebrae indicated if disc indicators are not present.

Disc Injuries to the Lower Back
(Radiating or Sciatic Pain and Weakness in the Hip, Leg, and Foot)

WHAT IS IT?

When people have severe back pain, the first thing they think is "slipped disc." In reality, only 2 percent of lower-back and leg pain is caused by disc problems, according to most doctors. Ligament injuries in the lower back and sacrum cause pain similar to that caused by disc injuries, and the two are frequently confused.

The discs that separate each of the vertebrae and act as shock absorbers in the spine can cause pain in two ways. A piece of the outer portion of the disc, which is made of hard fibrous tissue, can crack off and press against a sensitive spinal nerve. The other possibility is that the outer portion can split, allowing the central portion, which is softer and slightly pulpy, to ooze and protrude, causing pressure on a nerve. When a part of a disc presses on a nerve, pain can be felt in the back, hip, or down the leg and foot, depending on the referred pathway. Pain radiating down the thigh and lower leg is referred to as sciatic pain. The disc itself doesn't hurt: the pain comes from the nerve under pressure.

It is often difficult for the best of physicians to differentiate between disc and ligament problems in the back. What follows in this section are some guidelines to help you be as clear with your doctor as you can.

HOW AND WHY

The pain from a disc injury can come on in at least four different ways: (1) a sudden flash of pain, usually while lifting something heavy; (2) a gradual increase in pain over several days of hard physical work, or waking up with it the next morning after a heavy day of work; (3) a severe accident; or (4) a gradual appearance for no apparent reason whatsoever. The clearest distinguishing feature of a disc injury is a gradually increasing weakness of the mus-

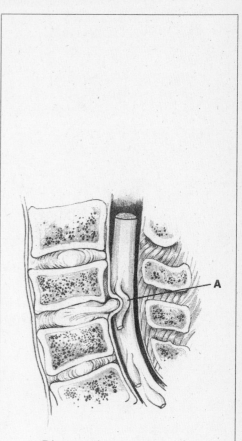

Disc pressing on a nerve (A)

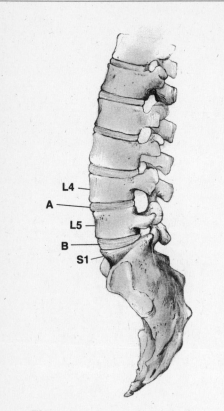

The most common disc injuries occur at A and B.

cles that control the foot, the thigh, or the buttock on one side of the body. The most obvious is when you lose control of the foot in walking. This is referred to as "foot drop." There are also pins-and-needle sensations sometimes, and a pronounced feeling of numbness. The tingling, numbness, or weakness are more decisive factors than the pain or its location, because the ligament tears in the sacrum can cause identical pain symptoms. Weakness occurs because the electrical impulses that tell your muscles what to do are gradually cut off by the constant pressure on a nerve. If the pressure is strong enough, pain will disappear completely as the weakness increases. The most common disc injuries occur to the bottom two discs at the levels L4–L5 (A) and L5–S1 (B).

There are many theories as to why discs rupture and cause so much pain, but in fact no one has any definitive answers. My own experience leads me to believe that some people are more prone to disc and ligament problems than others, based on their general health, both emotional and physical. In one family five of seven brothers required disc surgery. This suggests a hereditary factor also.

DIAGNOSTIC VERIFICATION

Diagnosing your own disc problems is very difficult and involves many tests for the strength of various muscles. This is too difficult to perform on yourself. See an orthopedist or a neurosurgeon, as this type of injury may require immediate medical attention. The most serious disc injury occurs when the nerve that controls bladder and bowel function is impinged upon. When urination and bowel functions are disturbed along with back and/or leg pain, a doctor should be seen immediately. If untreated, this type of disc problem can cause a permanent dysfunction in excretion, or paralysis. Fortunately, this rarely happens— but it is a good reason to be careful.

When disc surgery is contemplated a myelogram is often given in a hospital. Dye is injected into the spinal canal and an X ray is taken. This test is usually used only to confirm an already fairly positive diagnosis and is not reliable

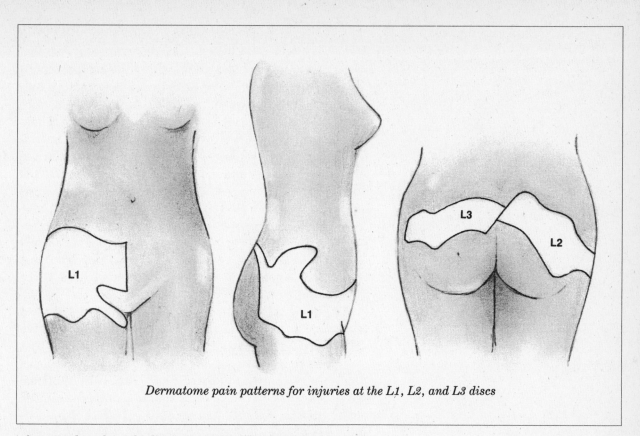

Dermatome pain patterns for injuries at the L1, L2, and L3 discs

when used as the only diagnostic tool. The dermatome patterns of pain here may help you to locate which disc is injured. See p. 248 also.

TREATMENT CHOICES

Self-Treatment

Some disc injuries heal themselves within nine to fifteen months. When a disc has protruded out of its encasement, it no longer receives any nourishment. It slowly dries and shrivels up and is then reabsorbed by the body. If you choose to wait, avoid activities that cause you pain, such as lifting heavy objects, and always lift things by bending your knees. Use a specially designed lower-back cushion, called the Posture Curve Lumbar Support Cushion, whenever you sit.* This supports your back in the proper posi-

*Relaxation Tools, Inc., P.O. Box 1045, New York, N.Y. 10025.

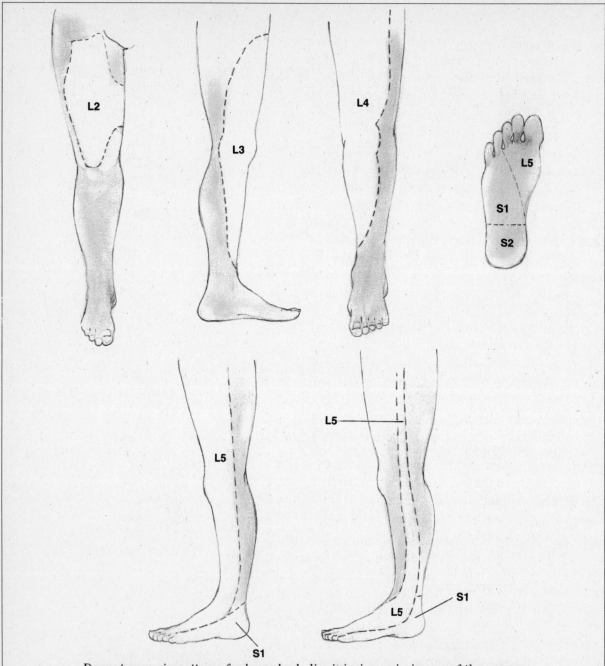

Dermatome pain patterns for lower-back disc injuries: pain in any of these areas probably means a disc injury at the level indicated by the number in the illustration.

tion and removes pressure from discs and ligaments. All this takes patience. Sometimes, if untreated, disc problems will remain for many years or a lifetime. Gravity guidance traction,* as described below, has proved to be effective in many cases.

Medical Treatment

1. TRACTION: In some cases of disc injuries the use of strong traction (between eighty and two hundred pounds) has been found to be very effective.† This traction is performed daily for one-half hour for up to two weeks.

2. GRAVITY GUIDANCE TRACTION PROGRAM: This is an intensive treatment program lasting up to one week, consisting of gravity guidance traction, hanging upside down, flexion and extension exercises, along with ultrasound and diathermy in severe cases. Dr. Robert Martin, the developer of this method, reports success in even severe cases.

3. EXERCISES: Many different systems of exercise claim great success. Although this has never been verified to everyone's satisfaction, they seem to work in some cases and not in others. I have seen them help people in many cases but have never known them to be long lasting. If they help it's a good idea to do them.

4. EPIDURAL INJECTION: This slowly given injection of anaesthetic into the spinal canal is amazingly effective in some cases. Safe and straightforward, it is also a good test to verify a disc injury. It will cause the pain to abate within five to ten minutes—and if it works the pain does not return.

5. CHYMOPAPAIN INJECTION: A newly developed treatment, this enzyme injection causes the disc to disintegrate, relieving pressure from the nerve. It is thought to be 80 percent effective in certain types of disc problems.

*Relaxation Tools, Inc.

†Cyriax and Russell, *Textbook of Orthopaedic Medicine*, vol. II (Baltimore, 1978).

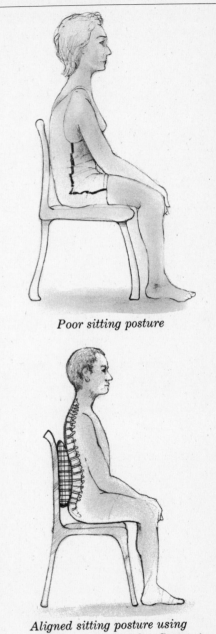

Poor sitting posture

Aligned sitting posture using Posture Curve Lumbar Support Cushion

6. SURGERY: A certain percent of disc injuries respond only to surgery. When a part of the disc is actually pressing strongly on a nerve and won't let up, it must be removed. There are risks in every operation and the possible dangers should be weighed against the benefits.

Rehabilitation
Do all back exercises that you can do without pain daily (pp. 272–76).

Sacral Ligament Tears

WHAT IS IT?

In the 1940s the buzzwords for lower-back pain were "Oh, my aching sacroiliac." In the fifties and sixties everything was slipped discs. Though the sacroiliac theory passed out of vogue, it was actually very accurate. Tears of sacroiliac and other ligaments of the sacrum account for a great majority of lower-back and so-called sciatic pain, but many physicians are unaware that the sacral area can cause such far-reaching problems. Tears of the sacroiliac ligaments (A) cause back pain, hip pain, and "sciatic" pain down the leg. These ligaments hold the sacrum to the hip bones, which are called ilia; hence, the sacroiliac ligaments. These ligaments hold together and help stabilize the back of the pelvis. They consist of thousands of individual fibers that are deeply layered for about an inch. They commonly cause pain across the very lowest part of the back (illustration on this page), down the thigh and lower leg.

Tears of the sacrotuberous and sacrospinous ligaments (B and C) cause referred pain only down the leg. Ligaments B and C hold the lower part of the sacrum to the bottom of the pelvis. Tears of these ligaments cause the pain patterns described below and illustrated on these pages.*

*Pain referred down one or both legs occurs in many different patterns: down the front thigh, in the outer lower leg, and so on. Here we show only the most common patterns.

The most common pain pattern for injuries to the sacroiliac ligaments

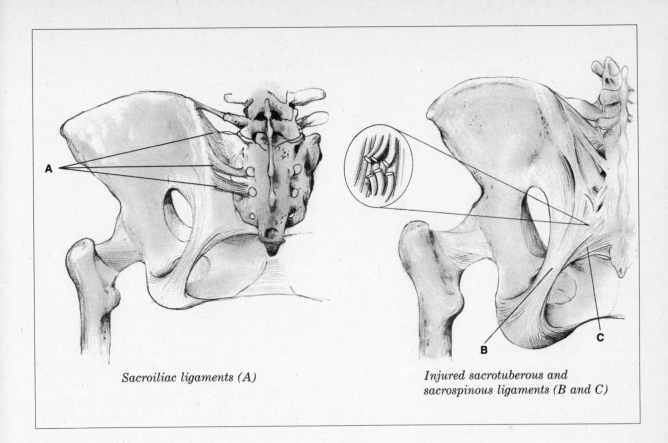

Sacroiliac ligaments (A)

*Injured sacrotuberous and
sacrospinous ligaments (B and C)*

HOW AND WHY

While the history of back pain may vary a great deal from
individual to individual, there seem to be four different
kinds of pain caused by tears of the ligaments in the sacrum. In each of the following categories pain may appear
either suddenly or slowly over the course of many hours.
It is also not uncommon to wake up with pain.

1. Periodically, severe back pain, with or without leg
pain, or leg pain alone, immobilizes the person. The pain is
intense and may come on after activity or prolonged sitting. The patient often takes to his bed and waits for the
pain to subside. This may take several days, a week, or a
month. The pain may for no reason disappear as suddenly
as it came, or it may lessen slowly, until the individual is
completely fine—that is, until the next attack.

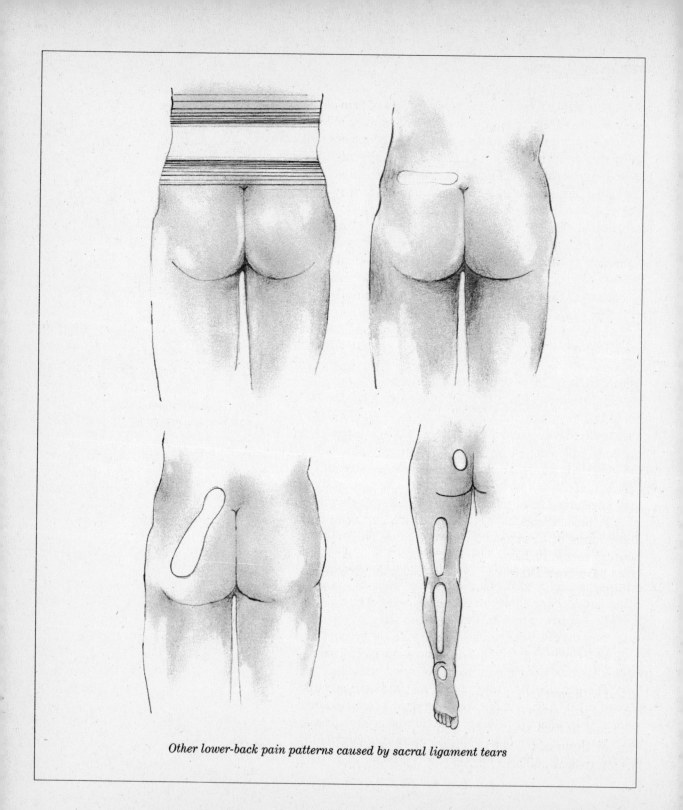

Other lower-back pain patterns caused by sacral ligament tears

2. The person experiences the same type of pain as described above, but it is not severe. It may appear once or twice a week or several times a month. It may be brought on by certain activities that he has learned to avoid—such as prolonged sitting, lifting heavy objects without bending the knees, or certain twisting motions. There may be a hint of discomfort much of the time, but it is only occasionally bothersome. Pain may be felt straight across the lower-back area or on one side, but the pain may switch from right to left, from episode to episode. One thinks of it more as a nuisance than as an actual injury, unless one day it changes to the kind of pain described in 1, 3, or 4.

3. The person becomes "fixed" in a bent position. He's in trouble. Frequently he is doubled up and cannot straighten. Sometimes the body is bent to the side, or twisted with one hip raised. There is constant muscle spasm and any attempt to straighten himself to a normal standing position causes excruciating pain. This may last for hours, days, or even longer, and usually abates slowly over many days. It is often a frightening experience, for the body feels immobilized and distorted.

4. Fairly intense back pain with or without leg pain, or just leg pain, is felt constantly for many many years. This may have come all at once or after experiences described in 1, 2, or 3. Drugs have usually been tried, along with many kinds of therapy, possibly including surgery, but nothing seems to help. The individual's life and mental state have been altered by the constant pain. There may be difficulty in sleeping and the person's spirit often appears broken, for this is indeed a difficult way to live.

DIAGNOSTIC VERIFICATION

Test

Stand with your feet together. Bend forward slowly, until you feel pain or an increase in pain. Do the same bending back and to each side. With sacral ligament injury, one, two, or three of these movements are usually painful in the lower-back and/or leg area.

When the ligaments of the sacrum are strained, the individual generally points right to the sacral ligaments. Discomfort is felt across the lowest part of the back and/or in the upper-hip region. In cases where there is only a pain in the leg, it is difficult to evaluate by yourself. The most telling thing is what is *not* present. When ligaments are torn there is no weakness, or pins and needles, as with a disc injury. There is just pain and sometimes a numblike sensation. The only way to be absolutely sure is to have the sacral ligaments injected with numbing medicine such as novocaine to see if the pain disappears. If it doesn't you have a disc or other ligament injury. Evaluating this yourself can be a tricky business.

TREATMENT CHOICES

Lower-back pain has plagued human beings for thousands of years and we still don't really understand the causes. There are carvings of traction devices from thousands of years ago. From everything we know, exercise shouldn't help injuries to these ligaments, but for some reason sometimes it does. If it helps, do it.

All of the treatments described below work some of the time, but certainly not in every case. The most success has been found with the use of proliferant injections. Sometimes the results are quite dramatic, relieving a great deal or all of the pain.

Self-Treatment

1. REST: Get some books and go to bed and rest for anywhere from a few days to a few weeks. This frequently permits the inflamed ligaments to heal, at least temporarily. If your back hurts only on athletic exertion or lifting, your rest period may just consist of not doing those activities.
2. EXERCISE: A daily exercise regimen for the lower back and abdominal muscles can reduce pain or keep it at bay. There are many books filled with exercise regimes, the most popular of which is *Backache, Stress*

and Tension* by Hans Kraus, M.D. Any physiotherapist can give you a set of back exercises. I have found these to be only temporarily effective, but some people swear by them.

Medical Treatment

1. MANIPULATION: Osteopathic and chiropractic manipulation often work to eliminate pain from overstressed sacral ligaments. One to five manipulations should be all that is necessary if this treatment is going to be effective. If it takes longer than that, you would probably do just as well by resting or waiting. No one knows exactly why the manipulation works, although there are many theories. One is that the sacrum has slightly dislocated itself, causing a constant pulling strain on the ligaments. The manipulation allows the sacrum to go back into place, thereby relieving the stress. Another theory is that it tears the strained fibers and when they heal they are stronger. Manipulation is frequently a good temporary solution.

2. TRACTION: Doctors frequently dispute how much traction should be used on lower-back injuries. Some say eighteen to twenty-five pounds constantly for weeks at a time. This, in my experience, is not terribly effective. In England, a method widely popularized by James Cyriax is the use of strong traction (eighty to two hundred pounds in proportion to body weight) daily for half an hour for up to two weeks. This treatment has a reasonably good success rate, but only for individuals with certain symptoms. This needs to be evaluated by a physician familiar with this method of traction. Again, why this works is not well understood.

3. INJECTION: Proliferant injections into the affected sacroiliac ligaments is the most effective treatment in the long run. This is because it promotes healing and

*(New York, 1975.)

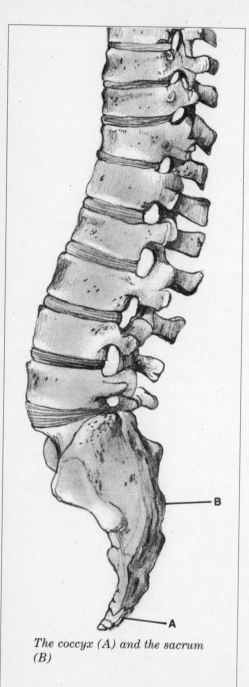

The coccyx (A) and the sacrum (B)

strengthening of the ligaments, which helps prevent the recurrence of this strain. Approximately six injections are usually needed, although sometimes half this number works. It is imperative that the doctor inject all the inflamed ligaments. This is why you need a number of visits. After each treatment the area of pain is usually smaller. The patient can then more easily guide the physician to the remaining areas of pain so that he can inject these.

Rehabilitation

Begin with Back Series 1. Later add Back Flexion and Back Lift. When feeling better add Back Series 2 (pages 272–76).

Tailbone Pain
(Coccygeal Ligament Tears)

WHAT IS IT?

It ain't no fun sitting down. It hurts like hell! This is one of the most miserable injuries you can get. When you injure your tailbone (coccyx), you've either strained the ligaments surrounding the coccyx or, in some cases, fractured the bone. You feel a sharp stabbing pain at the base of your spine when you sit down and possibly an ache in the lower spine when you're walking around. The coccyx (A) is a vestigial bone (it has no known function). If we were monkeys at one time, it was part of our tail. It's the last vertebra in our spine beneath the sacrum (B) and is surrounded by ligaments (C) which keep it in place.

HOW AND WHY

The world is full of practical jokers who think it's funny to pull chairs out from under you when you're about to sit down. There is nothing funny about it if you land on the floor and injure your coccyx. Severe falls are the cause of many injuries to the tailbone. Ice skaters and roller skaters injure their coccyx when they take a whopping fall.

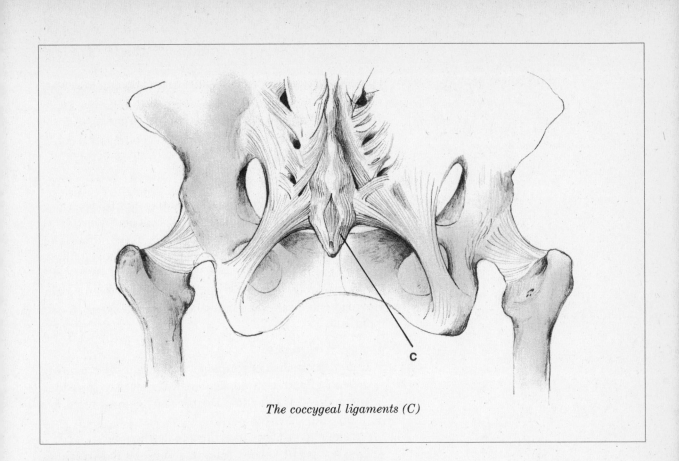

The coccygeal ligaments (C)

Martial arts enthusiasts are prone to the injury if they hit the ground wrong. I'm really sorry to report that it can also happen for absolutely no reason.

With this injury it's very difficult, if not impossible, to sit down on a hard chair or any hard surface. Something soft and spongy is a possible, but often uncomfortable, seat. Any pressure on the tailbone causes pain. If you've injured yourself severely, it hurts all the time. If you're only moderately injured, it hurts during vigorous activity as well as when you sit down; and in its mildest form you feel pain only when you sit down.

DIAGNOSTIC VERIFICATION

Test
If you have this injury it's pretty hard to miss, but to test for it you only need to put your fingers at the end of your

spine and press upward. In some cases bending backward causes pain as well. If you've fallen it's wise to see a physician and have an X ray to check for fractures.

TREATMENT CHOICES

Self-Treatment

It's called "wait!" While you're waiting, go to a surgical supply store and buy a doughnut. This is not to have with coffee, except indirectly. It's a round, firm rubber ring that keeps your tailbone suspended in the air, and it allows you to sit without your coccyx hitting the chair. Without it you'd probably have to drink your coffee standing up. Healing time can take anywhere from a week to six months.

Medical Treatment

1. INJECTION: Corticosteroid or proliferant injections are both effective in dealing with this injury, provided the physician can find the precise ligaments that are injured. This can sometimes be hard to do. It may take two or three injections to do the job.
2. SURGERY: In severe fractures surgery is sometimes performed and the coccyx is removed.

III.

13

Rehabilitation:
Getting Back on the Track

What is full recovery? It means you are as strong, coordinated, and flexible as you were before you were injured—anything less is not a full recovery, and in a partially recovered state you will be prone to injury again. There are two parts to recovery: rehabilitation and reconditioning. Rehabilitation means helping the injured part to heal and strengthening it for normal activity. While rehabilitating, all attention is *concentrated* on the injured part. Reconditioning, the second part of recovery, gets the injured area functioning well with the rest of the body. It requires increasing the strength and flexibility to levels needed for your normal activities as well as more taxing activities, such as athletics, dancing, and so forth. Another part of reconditioning is to re-establish a coordinated use of the body in which all body parts are carrying their fair share of the burden.

Recovery is never fun. Unfortunately, prevention seems like a good idea only after you've been injured. The one thing many people learn from their injuries is that they want and need a way to maintain their health so they

261

can avoid going through this ordeal again. They also learn to pay attention to early warning signals that announce that they are becoming vulnerable to injury.

TREATMENT

Treating your injury is the first step in rehabilitation and can be done alone or with outside help. Your treatment might consist of resting the injured part or applying ice to it. It might also entail seeking medical treatment, deep massage, or any of the appropriate treatments described in Chapter 5.

SELF-CARE

The first thing people ask after an injury is "How soon will I be better?" The answer is simple. We don't know but the better you take care of yourself, the faster your injury will heal. Taking care of yourself may mean taking lots of warm baths, or whirlpools, eating a good diet, taking vitamins if you need them, and getting plenty of sleep. Most healing occurs during the time you sleep. That's why people want to sleep more when they're sick.

As soon as you're able to do so without pain, you should begin moving the injured part of your body several times throughout the day, but be sure the movement is not too stressful. This will help reduce muscle atrophy and minimize the formation of scar tissue.

TENSION REDUCTION*

After an injury, you often find that the tension in your body has increased, especially in the injured area. This increase in muscle tension is a normal response to trauma, but when it is not discharged it can hamper proper healing. An excessive amount of muscular tension prevents the normal flow of blood and slows down the healing process. It does this by squeezing off the blood flow through

---

* Several of these types of exercises are given in Ben E. Benjamin, *Are You Tense?* (New York, 1978), and *Sports Without Pain* (New York, 1979).

small blood vessels. If you work to reduce the tension in your body, especially around the injured part, you will maximize the supply of oxygen and nutrients that promote the healing process. When the excess tension is released it's as though gates have opened and the blood can circulate freely to your injured area.

Warm baths, mentioned earlier, help to reduce tension. Deep massage, done by an accomplished professional, is also a very effective way of reducing tension levels. Gentle techniques, such as deep breathing and relaxation exercises, can also help to combat tension, as long as they don't cause you any pain.

STRENGTH RECOVERY

As soon as you are injured, atrophy begins. Atrophy is the breakdown of muscle, ligament, or tendon fibers as the result of disuse. The strength of muscles is lost at a very rapid rate as the muscle tissue shrinks in size. Tendons and ligaments are weakened by demineralization—the breakdown of their chemical composition. The longer the injury persists, the more the imbalance and atrophy continue. This sets the stage for further injury unless a rehabilitation and reconditioning program is followed faithfully. It is hard to imagine, but significant amounts of atrophy can occur in just a week or two.

Atrophy weakens the entire muscle-tendon unit. Since the strength and integrity of each fiber of the body is maintained by use, it is vitally important to move your body as much as possible without provoking pain during the recovery period. Even if you are consciously using your body, some atrophy usually occurs as a result of an injury. To counteract this it is important to rebuild your strength as soon as possible after your injury has healed.

STRENGTH BUILDING

The next question people ask is "Am I going to be strong again?" Yes! You can recover your strength in a number of ways through movement, isometric exercise, or the use of weights.

Let's say the muscle you want to rehabilitate is your front thigh. That muscle lifts the knee toward the chest and straightens the knee. In the movement approach you would do exercises such as knee-to-chest lifts, single-leg lifts with a straight knee, or running in place. In the isometric method you would place your hand on your knee and attempt to lift your leg against the resistance of your arm, hold it for ten seconds, and release. In the weight-training approach you would attach light weights, five to ten pounds, to your foot and lift your thigh or straighten your leg with five or ten repetitions in a row; or you might use an apparatus such as a Universal gym.

The use of light weights is what is generally recommended when you begin reconditioning, gradually increasing the weights to sixty to eighty pounds as your thigh gains strength.

ALIGNMENT

As we discussed on pages 22–23, the problem of alignment can often be a cause of injury, and restoring good alignment—so that there is a minimum of strain on your muscles, tendons, and ligaments—can play an important role in both recovering from and preventing injury. Often when you've been injured you begin to compensate by favoring the injured part for a brief period of time. When the pain has diminished, good alignment habits need to be re-established.

Though alignment problems are often subtle, there are some noticeable indicators of poor alignment, such as the head pushed way forward, the shoulders slumped with a collapsed chest, or shoulders raised and pulled back, an overly accentuated or flattened lower-back curve, turned-in knees, pronated or flat feet.

Pay attention to your alignment* as you begin activity again. If your foot-knee alignment is off, you may want to see a sports podiatrist, or see a movement specialist to

---

* For alignment tests and corrective exercises, see *Sports Without Pain*, chapters 5 and 9.

learn how to move in better alignment.* You can fall into poor alignment without realizing it. A young woman I worked with injured her hip, and in her attempt to ease her pain developed a habit of bending over when walking. For years after the injury, she was still walking in a stooped-over position that had become a habit. As a result, she had developed a chronic upper-back ache.

REHABILITATIVE EXERCISE

Rehabilitation is boring but necessary. It's boring because it involves the patient, tedious repetition of simple exercises. It's necessary to strengthen the injured area so that you can safely integrate it back into normal, active functioning. When is the right time to start rehabilitating? As soon as you can do the exercises without pain. Some people think that when you are injured you need to stay very still, but this is a misconception. The best healing is accompanied by movement. Movement prevents the formation of poor and unwanted scar tissue, and it minimizes the weakening caused by atrophy, which we discussed earlier in the chapter.

There are many different kinds of rehabilitative exercises that are effective. I have devised a set that can be done as part of an ice treatment, in which case they are started almost immediately. When you can move without pain you can do them independently. These are by no means the only rehabilitative exercises you can use, but they are simple and easy to do. Begin with five repetitions, or ten if five is too easy. Rest for thirty seconds between each set of five or ten. For instance: five, rest, five, rest, five, rest, etc., increasing by units of five every other day until you reach fifty; or if you wish to start at ten: ten, rest, ten, rest, etc., increasing by units of ten until you reach fifty to eighty. Do what seems easy and increase

* Movement specialists include practitioners of the Alexander technique; Bartinieff fundamentals; practitioners of the work of Lulu Sweigard, Barbara Clark, and the Benjamin system of muscular therapy.

very slowly. If you have pain or extensive soreness, drop back and increase at a slower rate.

When the use of weights is necessary for an exercise, begin with three or five pounds and work your way up to eight or ten pounds. If you are very strong, and accustomed to working with weights, you may want to go a little higher. These suggested weight levels apply to all the exercises except the thigh, where higher levels are given. Always use a weight that you are comfortable with and build up extremely gradually. When you advance to a heavier weight, drop the number of repetitions you are doing and begin building slowly again.

Foot, Ankle, Shin, and Calf Exercises

Your foot and ankle are controlled by your shin and calf muscles. This is why the rehabilitative exercises are the same for all these parts. For maximum rehabilitation it's best to do all of the exercises listed, but accent the exercises that directly work the area you have injured.

CIRCLES:
Sitting in a chair, cross your injured leg over your good one. Rotate your foot in as wide a circle as you can both clockwise and counterclockwise. Begin with ten circles in each direction. This is a particularly good exercise for injuries to the ankle.

ANKLE FLEXION:
Still sitting in a chair with your leg crossed, flex your ankle so your toes come toward your knee. Hold this for two seconds, now point your foot and hold that for two seconds too. Begin with five repetitions of flexing and pointing before resting. This is particularly helpful for injuries to the front and back of the foot and lower leg.

HEEL RAISES:
Stand and hold on to something beside you for balance. Without bending your knees, rise up onto the balls of your

feet. Keep your feet parallel. Stay there for a moment and come down again. Begin with five repetitions and then repeat this same exercise with the knees slightly bent. Bending the knees works a different muscle. If you've injured your Achilles tendon or calf, these exercises are especially important.

INNER-ANKLE LIFT:
For this exercise you'll need some props. You can either buy special weights that attach to the foot or you can use a small shopping bag, preferably plastic, with a five-pound weight, or cans that total five pounds, inside. Sitting in a chair, cross your injured leg over your good leg with either the weight apparatus or the loaded shopping bag across the front part of your foot just behind your toes, as illustrated. Now raise your foot toward the ceiling five or ten times, repeating after a rest. This exercise is good for injuries to the inner foot, ankle, or lower leg.

OUTER-ANKLE LIFT:
You need the same props for this exercise that you used in the Inner-Ankle Lift. Lie on your side on a couch with your knees bent (see p. 268). The injured foot or injured lower leg should be on top. Now extend the top leg off the edge of the couch or bed. Wearing the weight or the shopping bag, lift the outside of your foot toward the ceiling, keeping your foot pointed. Begin this exercise with ten repetitions. Do it again, but this time keep your foot flexed. This is a good exercise if you've injured the outer ankle and the outside of the lower leg.

Knee and Thigh Exercises

Many of the same exercises are good for rehabilitating the knee and thigh. Most injuries to the knee need either time or treatment to heal. Since certain thigh muscles control the movement of your knee, they often suffer and weaken as a result of knee injuries and therefore also need strengthening when your knee is injured.

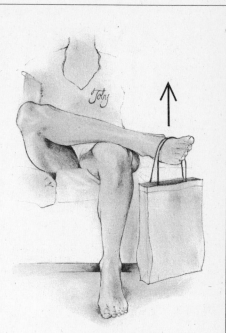

Inner-Ankle Lift

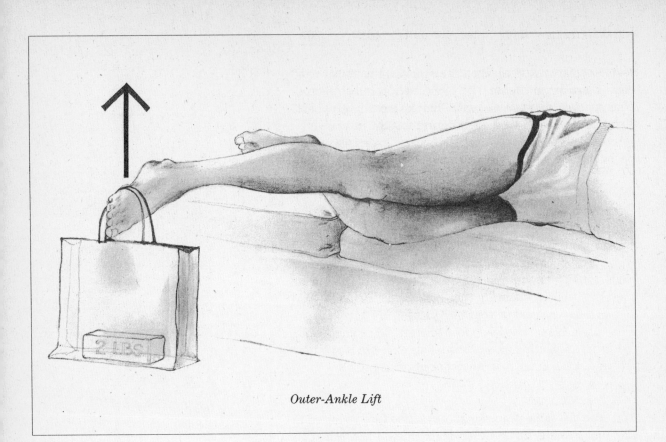

Outer-Ankle Lift

KNEE EXTENSION:
You need to have foot weights for this exercise, beginning with five pounds and working your way up to fifty or sixty pounds. Sit on a table with your legs dangling, wearing your weights. Slowly straighten your leg, hold it a moment, then lower it again. Repeat this ten times before resting and starting again. It may take four to six weeks to build up to maximum weight. This exercise is good for rehabilitation after knee injuries, particularly after patella tendinitis.

THIGH LIFT:
Again sit on a table so your foot doesn't touch the ground. You can do this exercise with or without foot weights.

Keeping your back fairly erect, raise and lower your thigh ten times. Do it with the leg bent and later on with it straight. Rest and repeat again. This exercise is good for injuries to the front thigh and the front of the hip.

UP, OUT, IN, DOWN:
Sit in a chair with your knees bent. Raise your foot about three inches off the ground, straighten your leg out in front of you, bend your leg again, then replace it on the floor. Start with five repetitions. Injuries to the front knee and front thigh are especially helped by this exercise.

SIDE-LYING LIFT:
Lie on your side with your knees slightly bent, keeping the injured leg on top. With your knee bent, very slowly raise your leg about a foot in the air, then slowly lower it. Start with five repetitions. This exercise is good for injuries to the outer thigh.

THIGH SQUEEZE:
Sitting in a chair, place a ball between your knees. Squeeze the ball for five seconds at a time and repeat three times before resting. This exercise helps inner-thigh injuries.

HAMSTRING STRENGTHENERS:
Lie face down, keeping your body flat and your legs straight. Lift your injured leg into the air as high as you can, keeping your knee *straight*. Begin with five or ten repetitions. Lying in the same position with weights attached to your foot, bend your knee and lift your foot toward the ceiling so that your leg makes a 90° angle. Begin this with ten repetitions. Both of these exercises strengthen the hamstrings and can be done separately or together.

Elbow and Forearm Exercises

The muscles and tendons of the forearm are responsible for most injuries to the elbow. Begin these exercises with

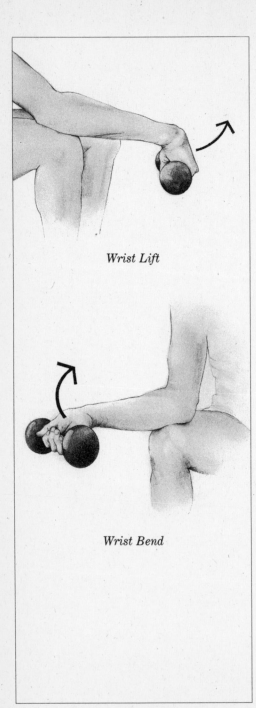

Wrist Lift

Wrist Bend

a three- or five-pound weight and work your way up to eight or ten pounds.

WRIST LIFT:
Sit in a chair and rest your elbow on your knee. Hold the weight in your hand with your palm facing the floor, as shown. Lift your wrist as far up as it will go, then slowly bring it back to its original position. Begin with five or ten repetitions, slowly increasing the weight when you have reached fifty repetitions. As you increase the weight, lower the number of repetitions and rebuild them slowly again. This is good for outer-forearm pain and tennis elbow.

WRIST BEND:
This exercise is the same as above, except that you turn your arm over so your palm faces the ceiling. This is good for inner-forearm strains and golfer's elbow.

Shoulder and Upper-Arm Exercises

To do all of the following exercises you should have weights ranging from three to ten pounds. If you are very strong you may need a heavier one.

FOREHAND LIFT:
A) Lie on your back on the floor with your arm bent at the elbow. Keep your upper arm against your body. Allow your forearm to fall outward so that your hand almost touches the floor. In this position grip your weight and very slowly bring your forearm straight up into a vertical position, then slowly lower it again. Begin this exercise with ten repetitions.

B) Still lying on the floor, extend your arm straight above your head and let it rest on the floor. Gripping the weight very slowly, raise your arm until it is vertical. Slowly lower it back to the original position above your head and start again. Do only five repetitions of this exercise to start. Both these exercises work the subscapularis muscle-tendon unit, which is used in forehand and throwing.

BACKHAND LIFT:

Again lie on the floor on your back and drop your forearm across your belly. Gripping the weight, slowly raise your forearm to a vertical position and then slowly lower it back across your belly. Begin with ten repetitions.

Now stand up. Lift your upper arm out to the side and let your lower arm hang scarecrow style. Gripping the

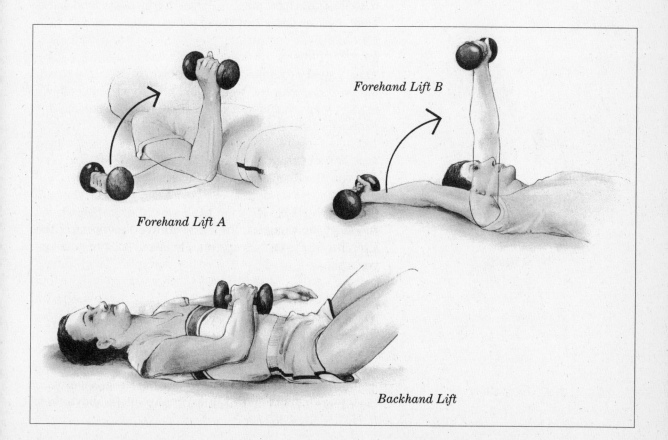

Forehand Lift A

Forehand Lift B

Backhand Lift

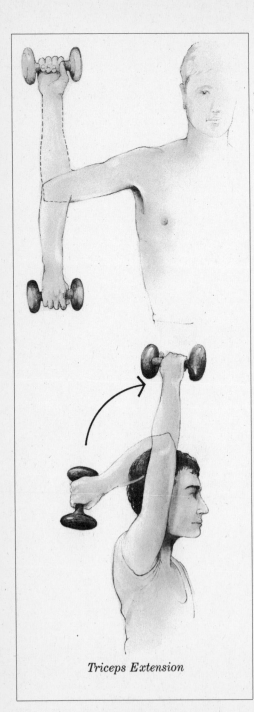

Triceps Extension

weight, lift your lower arm until your fist points to the ceiling, then lower it. Begin with ten repetitions. These two exercises work the muscle you use in backhand, the infraspinatus.

WEIGHTED ARM CIRCLE:
Stand up with a weight in your hand and move your arm out three to four inches from your body. Make a big, slow circle that crosses in front of your body, being careful not to bend your elbow. The error that people frequently make is to let the arm fall back behind the shoulder as it goes around. Try not to do this. Do five slow circles in each direction before taking a rest. This exercise is good for rehabilitating most shoulder injuries. It works the suitcase muscle, the supraspinatus, plus the forehand and backhand muscles described above.

BICEPS CURL:
This is a very common weight-lifting exercise. In a standing position, grip the weight and bring your hand slowly toward your shoulder. Do ten repetitions to begin. This exercise works the biceps.

TRICEPS EXTENSION:
You can stand or sit for this one. Holding the weight, extend your arm straight above your head. Keeping your upper arm vertical, let your hand slowly drop behind you toward your shoulder. To start, do five repetitions. This exercise works the triceps muscle in the back of your upper arm.

Back Exercises

There are dozens of back exercises, but there is a lot of controversy about how effective they are and what they can do. My sense is that their value lies in keeping your back more mobile and healthy. If any of these exercises hurt, DO NOT do them.

BACK SERIES 1:

This first series is quite gentle and is all done on your hands and knees. Your hands should be shoulder width apart and your knees four or five inches apart. Slowly rock your body forward (1) and back (2), going only four to six inches in each direction. Now rock your entire body side to side (3), shifting your weight from one arm and leg to the other. Don't let your head drop—keep it in line with your spine.

Round your center back up toward the ceiling, allowing your head and pelvis to come toward each other (4). Now slowly go the other way until your back is arched and you are looking straight ahead (5). Do each set about five times continuously, alternating the sets for two to three min-

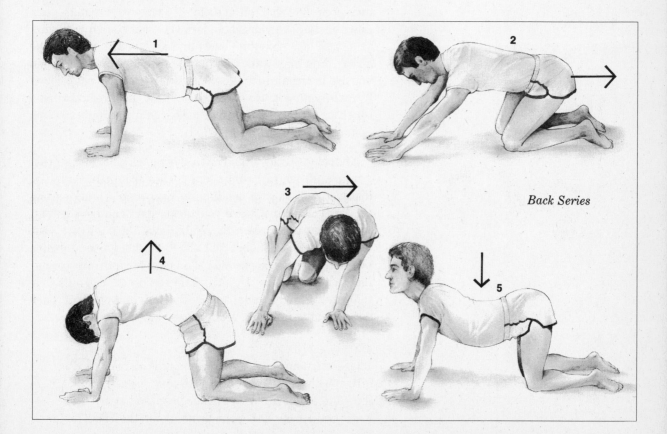

Back Series

utes. This series relaxes your back and enhances its mobility.

BACK SERIES 2—EXTENSION:
The back moves in essentially two directions, forward and back, and it's important to keep yourself mobile in both these directions. Most people do a lot of bending forward but rarely bend back. Begin with only a few of each of these back-extension exercises if they are difficult for you. If they hurt don't do them. Add only one or so more every other day. Start by holding each position three or four seconds, with the goal of holding each for ten seconds. The maximum number of times to do each exercise is six.

Press-up Arch: Lie on your back with your knees bent and your feet flat on the floor. Place your hands palm down just above your shoulders (1). Press down with your arms and legs simultaneously and arch your body into the air (2). You may want to adjust your hands and feet when you are in the air to make the position easier to hold. Slowly lower yourself. If your hands slip let them rest against a couch or a wall. If this one makes you uncomfortable in your knees or your back, skip it.

Standing Arch: Stand with your back to a wall so that you are fifteen to twenty-four inches from the wall. The distance will vary depending on your height and flexibility. Put your arms above your head and bend back so that your palms touch the wall. Walk down the wall with your hands as far as comfort will allow and hold a comfortable position for several seconds. You may have to adjust your feet to add stability. Be sure you keep breathing—it's easy to forget. Slowly walk back up the wall and push off, back to a standing position. If it causes pain, don't do it.

BACK FLEXION
There are many exercises that make the back flexible in a forward direction, but this is the easiest one I know. Sit on the edge of a chair with your legs spread apart. Bend forward and reach with your arms under the chair as far as

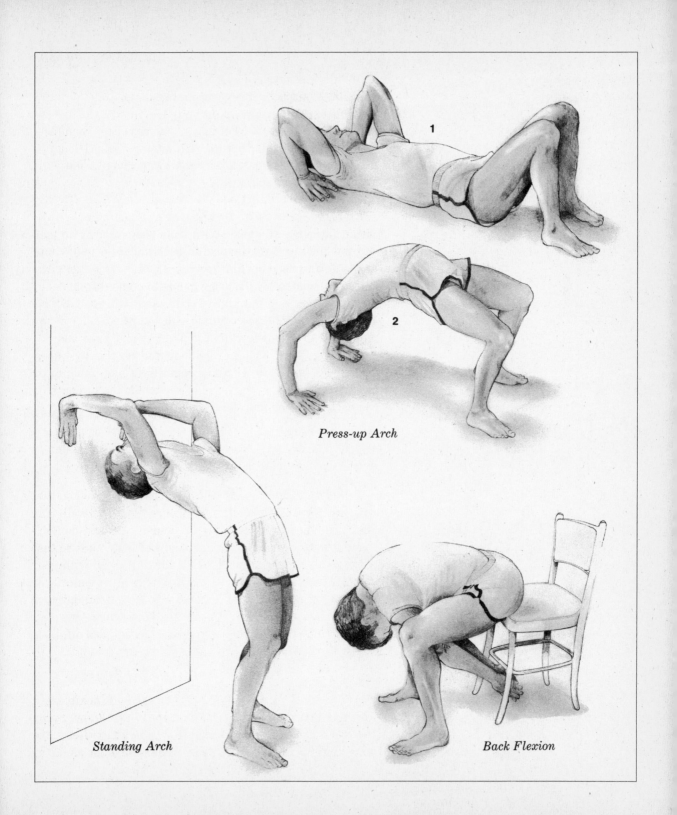

1

2

Press-up Arch

Standing Arch

Back Flexion

you can. Don't hold this position, but go up and down in a continuous motion, dropping your head and exhaling every time you go down. Do this in a series of ten, completing fifty or one hundred at each sitting. Take it easy—don't force it. This is an exercise often given along with proliferant injection therapy.

BACK LIFT

Sit on the edge of a chair with your legs spread two feet apart. Curve and relax your back and head, placing your hands on the floor in front of you. Slowly straighten your back and head, allowing your hands to come off the floor. Depending on your flexibility, your hands will probably be about a foot off the floor. Hold the lifted position for a moment and then slowly round your back and head and return to the floor. The more slowly you do this the more effective it is. Begin with five repetitions and build up to twenty or twenty-five. This exercise builds the strength of the back and neck muscles.

14

Reconditioning

Once you have rehabilitated the injured part of your body, you can begin to design a conditioning program to prepare yourself to re-enter more strenuous activity. Reconditioning means re-establishing the coordinated use of your body, getting your strength up to a level where you can safely enter athletic activity, and stretching out muscles that have lost their flexibility. This is a crucial part of any recovery program. Unfortunately, just because the injured part feels better, it doesn't mean that you are ready to rush into full-scale activity. If, in your impatience to get back to your activity again, you skip this period of adjustment, you are likely to end up with the same injury or a new one.

SWIMMING
Swimming is one of the best reconditioning activities. It is good cardiovascular exercise and will help you return to your activity with more endurance in the heart and lungs. Swimming encourages a coordinated use of almost every muscle in your body. You use your arms, legs, torso, and

head. It is also one of the safest forms of exercise because your body is weightless in the water. In this weightless state, the body does not have to absorb shock and can exercise with a minimum of stress.

For certain injuries, especially in the legs and feet, swimming can be started early in the rehabilitation phase, if it doesn't cause discomfort. The sooner you can start, the more you can avoid loss of muscular and cardiovascular strength.

STRENGTHENING

In reconditioning you are returning to the full physical capability you had prior to being injured. If your period of inactivity and rehabilitation was lengthy, you may need to rebuild the muscle strength in many parts of your body. The best way for you to begin a strength-reconditioning program is to re-enter slowly the sports or activities you were active in before you were injured. I would like to stress the word *slowly*, as this re-entry approach requires consistency and patience. If you were a runner who ran five miles a day before your injury, you can't hope to begin running this distance again as soon as you feel better. For the safest return to activity you would begin running every other day and slowly increase the distances, taking about a month to reach the full five miles.

Tennis players, in beginning to recondition, should start strengthening by volleying against a wall or with a friend for increasing periods of time. However, it would be a mistake to jump back into a competitive game before you have recovered your full strength. Competition is exciting and in your zeal you could easily push your limits to a dangerous point.

If you have regularly enjoyed taking exercise or dance class, begin by giving yourself short classes at home before you re-enter a class in which you may feel a pressure to keep up.

A useful adjunct in regaining your strength more rapidly is moderate weight training. If you are unfamiliar with using weights, it would be wise to consult a physical therapist or weight-training specialist for help in designing a weight program.

A helpful device I have recently discovered for both warm-up and reconditioning of the lower body is a small portable trampoline that can easily be used in your home.* These trampolines are very useful because they permit you to exercise vigorously while absorbing the stress to your muscles and joints.

An important component of reconditioning is warming up. Though it is easy to rationalize skipping this step, a thorough warm-up of ten to fifteen minutes should precede every strength-building workout. Why warm-ups are important will be explained more fully in the next chapter on prevention. The amount of time required to recoup completely your former capabilities depends on the severity of your injury and the length of time you were inactive.

WATER EXERCISES

Other kinds of exercises can be done in the water—for instance, walking or running in waist-deep water or jumping or leg lifts in deeper water. The advantage of water exercise is that you can work your muscle without putting weight or stress on it.

STRETCHING

People, like cats, feel the need to stretch. The function of stretching is to train the muscle fibers to remain in a more lengthened position and to decrease small amounts of tension that accumulate during strenuous activity. If your leg has been injured, or if you have not been able to use your legs as a result of an injury elsewhere, you will probably need to stretch for a while to regain the flexibility of your muscles. Many people confuse stretching with warming up, but they are separate and distinct activities.

---

* These small, round trampolines are six inches tall and three feet across. They are built so you don't bounce too high. The best-built model I've seen is the Sundancer.

HOW TO STRETCH

You can't stretch effectively if your body is not warmed up. When your muscles are cold, they resist stretching. Warmed-up muscles elongate and stretch easily and with very little discomfort. You will get the most benefit from stretching if you do it while sitting or lying down, without pushing or forcing. The goal is to stretch the muscles, not the tendons or ligaments. Tendons and ligaments become permanently damaged if you stretch them more than a very small amount. You can tell if you are stretching a tendon or ligament by paying attention to precisely where you feel the pulling sensations when you stretch. You should feel the pull in the central meaty part of the muscle

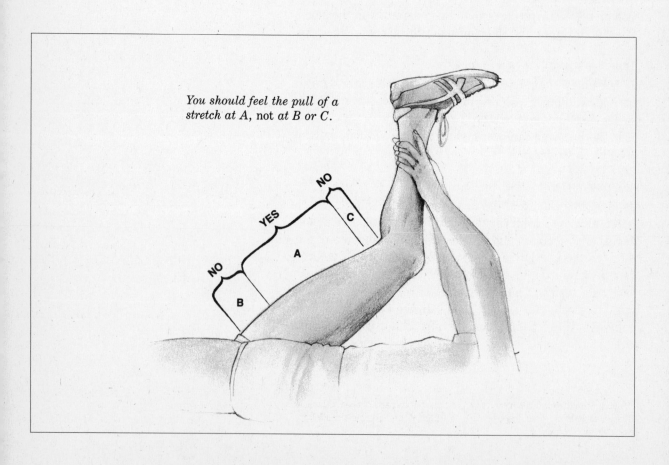

You should feel the pull of a stretch at A, not at B or C.

(A). If you feel the stretch near or over a joint, you are stretching a ligament or a tendon (B or C). If the stretch is felt in the wrong place when stretching the back thigh or calf area, you may need to bend your knee an inch or two during the stretch. Not all stretches suit your body, so if some make you uncomfortable, find others. The most important areas to keep stretched out are the calves, the hamstrings of the back thigh, the front thigh muscles, and, in some cases, the inner thigh.* You need only one or two good stretches for each part of the body, so doing many different ones really isn't necessary. To stretch effectively, hold each stretch for thirty to sixty seconds while relaxing and breathing deeply. Then rest for a moment between each stretch. An effective stretching session need take no longer than eight to ten minutes.

When using stretching as part of a reconditioning program, you will get the best results by stretching five or six times a week.

Some popular stretches that should be avoided, such as the plow and shoulder stand, can make you vulnerable to injury if practiced regularly over a period of time. They weaken the ligaments at the back of the neck. The hurdler's stretch, fourth position on the floor in dance, and the lotus position stress the knee ligaments in an unnatural way and weaken their structure. Also, if you place your leg up on a bar or table to stretch the hamstrings, you may overstress the tendons instead of stretching the muscle.

* See my *Sports Without Pain* (New York, 1979) for stretching exercises.

15

Prevention: Staying on the Track

Injury prevention is a book in itself—in fact, I wrote such a book—so here we will cover it only briefly. The ideal way to prevent injury is to be very conscious of your physical fitness: eat a balanced diet, get enough rest, keep your muscles relaxed and resilient, and exercise and stretch regularly.

Getting in shape is one thing. *Keeping* yourself in shape requires exercising regularly—three or four times a week, with a thorough warm-up beforehand and some stretching afterward—and learning and maintaining good alignment, especially in sports activity.

There are unavoidable injuries—freak accidents that we hear about all the time. In these cases, even being in good shape makes little difference. However, the vast majority of injuries can be prevented. You will probably have to make a conscious effort to learn new habits, but this will pay off within a short period of time.

DANGER SIGNALS

Out bodies send warning signals, coded messages. Sometimes we don't understand them. Other times we ignore them. One of the most common warnings is simply feeling "out of it." This can happen very subtly. Suddenly you're just daydreaming or drifting, your vision gets a little fuzzy, or you're feeling tired. These are all messages that it's time to stop.

There are many other warning signals: waking up sore and stiff, cramps in your legs, sudden sharp pains or a persistent headache. Listen to them. Your body is saying, "I need rest," "I need to slow down," or "I need some pampering. A massage or warm bath or a swim would be nice." To push forward when your body is asking you to slow down will increase your chance of injury.

GOOD EQUIPMENT

Saving money on cheap equipment can be very expensive. Quality equipment is more durable and safer. Buy the best when it comes to ski equipment, roller skates, ice skates, and football gear. Also be fussy about the fit. Don't let yourself be talked into something that doesn't feel good.

TENSION REDUCTION

Excess muscle tension has become as prevalent in our society as the common cold. Many of us have become so accustomed to living with very tense muscles that we don't even realize that they could relax. Suddenly, after a massage, a whirlpool, or a sauna, we realize that our body does feel different, and we understand how tense we usually are.

There are ways of maintaining lower levels of body tension, whether that extra tension is caused by emotional or physical stress. You can help your body relax and remain more resilient and supple through special relaxation techniques, such as deep breathing, biofeedback, relaxation tapes, or regularly scheduled deep massage. Another way to relieve excess tension is through impact exercises, such as hitting a punching bag or kicking a pillow around.

STRENGTH MAINTENANCE

Building your strength is different from maintaining your strength. For optimal prevention you need to maintain your strength through regular exercise or athletic activity. It's important to remember that your body loses its strength quickly. If you ski avidly all winter but don't exercise your legs during the rest of the year, you can't expect them to be as strong at the start of the next season. The same is true for all seasonal sports. Maintaining your strength is a year-round project.

WARM-UP

Warming up does just what the name implies. It increases blood circulation so that your muscles get hot—which makes them more pliable and more able to absorb shock. It entails a slow, progressive series of exercises, lasting from ten to fifteen minutes, depending on your body's needs, and it gradually increases your breathing and heart rates so that the oxygen supplied to your muscles is at its maximum. If your heart is not warmed up you will tire much more quickly and actually put a strain on the heart muscle. Stretching does not warm you up. Only exercises that contract the muscles can produce heat and directly affect blood circulation. For instance, slowly pointing and flexing your foot will warm up your lower leg: stretching your calf or shin muscles in the proper way will not.

Warming up should be geared toward the activity you are going to perform. Most activities involve the legs, so they should always get a warm-up. Additional exercises should be added for the arms when you are preparing for an upper-body sport, or sports that use both the upper and lower body equally.

Ideally, in all warm-ups you should begin while lying on the floor. You should warm up your joints first, and lying down allows you to do this without having your joints bear the weight of your body. Moderate strength-building exercises are used for the best warm-up.* Starting with the feet and legs, the exercises should slowly become more vigorous and include more and more parts of the body. Half of the warm-up should be done while standing and end with running in place for several minutes. For the most efficient warm-up, you should not have too much repetition of the same movement.

When warming up, alternating legs and body parts is important. It allows for the oxygen recovery needed by your muscles. If you have a short distance to travel to the field or courts, you can do a floor warm-up at home and the rest when you reach your destination.

Lastly, you want to warm up for your specific activity: practicing your shots on the racquetball court, volleying before a tennis game, throwing the ball for a while before softball, or doing some dance techniques before a class.

To some people a warm-up is a nuisance and they skip it or rush through it. Preventing injury takes effort; a good warm-up will prevent 50 percent of the injuries that occur. Not only will you suffer fewer injuries, but you will perform better as well, and because you are more supple you may be freer of the silent fear of injury that can hold you back from your full potential.

IN CONCLUSION

Much as I wish it could do so, I'm sure this book has not answered all of your questions about the aches and pains and injuries you can sustain as an active person. However, I hope it has given you many of the answers you have sought about

---

*See *Sports Without Pain*, chapters 3 and 4, for a thoroughly detailed warm-up.

what you might have done to yourself, or how or why you did it—or at least pointed you in the direction of finding those answers. Over a period of seven years I rewrote this book three times; each time the new information I learned and wanted to add amounted to a totally revised book. What you have just read has stood the test of three more years of investigation, and I feel confident in having presented it to you. I hope it will get you back on the track—or the court, or the slopes, or on stage, or in the saddle. I wish you a speedy recovery.

Appendix

Injection Manual for Physicians

Introduction to Injection Therapy for Musculoskeletal Injuries

Excessive inflammatory response to injury can result in disabling scarring with loss of muscle, tendon, and joint function. Adrenal cortical steroids used in moderation will control the inflammation and permit normal healing. Because excessive use of steroids will actually prevent healing of tissue and will produce atrophy, the frequency of injection must be carefully limited. Delayed healing resulting from repeated local injury with scar-tissue formation will respond to a local injection of a tissue irritant and accelerate healing. Three types of tissue stimulants are in use today. Sclerosants date back to 1835 and have been used for a variety of conditions. Inguinal hernias, varicose veins, and joint ligaments have responded to sclerosant injection by successful repair through scar-tissue formation. Since the 1950s, a modified sclerosant containing dextrose has been used in Germany and England. A doctor in Germany used sterile 10 percent pure dextrose in a local anaesthetic, while the English physicians added phenol and glycerine to the dextrose and American doctors used phenol and propylene glycol in stock solutions to permit storage for periods of time before use. The dextrose is a means of introducing a sterile hypertonic solution that is in greater concentration than the normal 0.10 percent concentration in the circulating blood. The osmotic pressure of 8 percent or 4 percent dextrose injected into the muscles, tendons, ligaments, and periosteum or synovial space increases the fluid content in areas injected until a balance is reached between the concentration in the space and that in the surrounding tissue. Attracted to the area of concentrated dextrose are the leukocytes and the macrophages in the circulating blood and surrounding tissues. These, in combination with the local inflammatory reaction, change a chronic condition to a temporarily acute condition with rapid repair of the injured tissues. The difference between pure dextrose and a typical sclerosant is that the sclerosant produces tissue destruction to a sufficient degree for scar formation with dense nonelastic connective tissue. This can be seen in histological studies of the action of sclerosant on muscle and connective tissue. The end result of pure dextrose injection in concentrations of up to 10 percent into rat muscle has failed to demonstrate any evidence of scar-tissue formation. The ideal of prolotherapy is to enhance repair without formation of scar tissue.

A physician in Pennsylvania and one in New York began to use pure dextrose in local anaesthetic in 1975 with much less local reaction and consistent improvement in musculoskeletal injuries of their patients. All solutions are sterile, and 70 percent ethyl alcohol is used to maintain sterility of the rubber-stoppered vials of dextrose solution in local anaesthetic.

"Trigger points" will be used as the descriptive term for sites of injury or inflammation that may refer pain to other areas. Trigger points are described as occurring in muscles with local fibrositis, in injured tendons, ligaments, and periosteal attachments to bone. Some of these are true trigger points in that they evoke a referred-pain syndrome to the dermatome levels in the skin and soft tissues at a distance from the point of pressure. Injection of inflammatory areas with corticosteroids can be followed by local infiltration of dextrose in local anaesthetic one to two weeks later. The proliferative response is the aim of treatment by prolotherapy. In the following section on injection technique, I will describe methods of treating acute and chronic musculoskeletal injuries.

Injection of small amounts of solution at close intervals as a series of dots is called stippling. Extensive areas of muscle attachment or tendon substance cannot be adequately treated with a single large amount of dextrose lidocaine. Stippling will permit identification of the areas of maximum sensitivity and inflammation.

A. Gale Borden, M.D.

The Foot and Ankle

Posterior Tibialis Tendinitis

INJURY:

Inflammation of the posterior tibial tendon and sheath occurs during uncontrolled strong plantar flexion of the foot and ankle with marked plantar pressure at the end of the range of flexion. Dancers and runners injure this tendon frequently.

SIGNS:

Marked tenderness over the posterior tibial tendon behind the medial malleolus and pain on plantar flexion of the ankle are present, along with pain on resisted inversion. In extreme cases, there is pronounced swelling.

TECHNIQUE:

Have the patient supine with the injured foot and ankle externally rotated. Feel behind the medial malleolus with a fingertip and follow the tendon proximally in its sheath and distally under the arch. Inject 5 mg prednisolone in 2 ml lidocaine into the tendon sheath and fill it if possible. After three minutes, test for tenderness and ability to jump and land on the affected foot. Repeat injection if further tender areas are still present. (See Fig. 1.)

Second Visit: Repeat treatment in one week if not completely pain free.

Effectiveness: Fifty percent are "cured" with one injection. Ninety percent of the rest will respond to a second treatment. In resistant cases, look for gout or pseudo-gout.

Anterior Tibialis Tendinitis

INJURY:

Overstretching or sudden stress will subject the tendon or its attachment to elongation beyond the physical limit and rupture some fibers. Sometimes the tendon of insertion is injured at the base of the first metatarsal bone and first cuneiform. Compression or friction may produce inflammation.

SIGNS:

Pain and tenderness occur along the course of the tendon where it is injured. Sometimes local swelling accompanies inflammation. Resisted dorsiflexion will reproduce the pain.

TECHNIQUE:

With the patient supine, locate the area of tenderness and apply povidone iodine. Fill a 5-ml luer-lock syringe with 5 mg prednisolone in 1 percent lidocaine and fit it with a sharp ⅝-inch 25-gauge cannula. Very gently penetrate the skin over the area of pain or swelling and infiltrate around the tendon with 1 or 2 ml suspension until it is free of pain. Test for efficacy by having the patient dorsiflex at the ankle. If no pain or tenderness is present, treatment is adequate. Tendon attachments to bone require injection with 8 percent dextrose in 1 percent lidocaine at the points of tenderness using 0.1-ml increments until pain free. Inject the tendon at the periosteal attachment sparingly. Do not overtreat.

Second Visit: Repeat the indicated treatment if disability continues. Caution against overuse after injection.

Effectiveness: Usually two injections will afford lasting relief. Some patients will resume full activity too early because of the absence of pain.

Peroneal Tendinitis

INJURY:

Inflammation within the tendon sheath can occur in the peroneus longus and brevis tendons behind the lateral malleolus. In addition, the peroneus longus has a tendon sheath in the sole of the foot where inflammation owing to excessive tension and compression can occur.

SIGNS:

Pain, local tenderness, and pain on resisted flexion with eversion of the foot is present behind the lateral malleolus or posterior to the base of the fifth metatarsal bone as the longus tendon travels beneath the cuboid bone.

TECHNIQUE:

Fill a 5-ml luer-lock syringe with 5 mg prednisolone in 1 percent lidocaine. Have the patient lying on the uninjured side and mark the areas of local tenderness with povidone iodine. With one fingertip on the tendon, inject the sheath proximally or distally with a sharp 1.5-inch 25-gauge cannula using 1 ml at a time until the tendon and tendon sheath are pain free. An injection into the sheath will relieve the inflammation in both tendons.

Second Visit: Within one week, repeat the treatment as necessary.

Effectiveness: Good results are usually obtained with this treatment.

Extensor Digitorum Longus Tendinitis

INJURY:

Inflammation of this tendon is frequent in dancers and runners.

SIGNS:

Pain, tenderness, and sometimes swelling will occur over the course of this tendon.

TECHNIQUE:

With the patient supine and the toes in strong dorsiflexion, palpate the tendon extending to the lateral four toes with one fingertip to find the area of tenderness. Mark with povidone iodine and fill a 3-ml syringe with 5 mg prednisolone in 1 percent lidocaine. Using sharp ⅝-inch 25-gauge cannula, inject directly into the subcutaneous area around the tendon with increments of 1 ml suspension. Keep the point well superficial to the dorsalis pedis artery. Treat until no pain or tenderness is present. Caution the patient to avoid any local pressure on this area.

Second Visit: Repeat this treatment after one week if necessary.

Effectiveness: Rapid improvement follows treatment. Two treatment visits are usually enough.

Extensor Hallucis Longus Tendinitis

INJURY:

Compression, friction, and excessive resistive motion will produce tendon inflammation.

SIGNS:

Local pain, tenderness, and especially pain on dorsiflexion of the great toe are present.

TECHNIQUE:

With the patient supine and the great toe in strong dorsiflexion, palpate the elevated tendon with one fingertip to find the tender area. Mark with povidone iodine and fill a 3-ml syringe with 10 mg prednisolone in 1 percent lidocaine. Using a sharp ⅝-inch 25-gauge cannula, inject directly into the subcutaneous area around the tendon with increments of 1 ml suspension. No pain on motion and no tenderness should be present after injection. Caution the patient to avoid constricting bandages and tight laces across this area.

Second Visit: Usually one injection is adequate, but a second treatment may be given after one week.

Effectiveness: This tendon readily responds to treatment and normal activity is possible within two weeks.

Great Toe Joint Pain

INJURY:

Compression of the metatarsophalangeal joint or the interphalangeal joint will produce acute synovitis. Gout with uric acid crystal formation, and osteoarthritis will also cause acute synovitis.

SIGNS:

Pain, swelling, and tenderness with loss of joint motion are present. Extreme passive flexion and extension are both painful.

TECHNIQUE:

If the metatarsophalangeal joint is disabled, gently move the joint to differentiate between the border of the base of the phalanx and the metatarsal head. Mark this with povidone iodine and fill a 3-ml luer-lock syringe with 10 mg prednisolone in 2 ml 1 percent lidocaine. Use a sharp ⅝-inch 25-gauge cannula and penetrate the skin anteromedially at the joint line. Inject 0.2 ml suspension and slowly penetrate the dense fibrous joint capsule. A sudden lack of resistance will indicate the joint space. Slowly fill the joint until it feels moderately distended. Withdraw the cannula and gently obtain maximum joint motion. The interphalangeal joint is less often injured. Inject this from an anterior approach at the medial border of the extensor tendon and use 0.5 ml steroid suspension.

Second Visit: Usually a single injection is adequate. Repeat the treatment after one week if pain continues.

Effectiveness: Treatment of gout with medication will prevent recurrence after infection. Traumatic synovitis usually responds to one treatment.

Plantar Fasciitis

INJURY:

Crush injury to the fascia extending from os calcis over the conjoined flexor tendon of the digitorum brevis is soon followed by inflammation. The fascia overlying the medial calcaneal tubercle and attached soft tissues is more often injured than that connected to the lateral calcaneal tubercle.

SIGNS:

Pain, tenderness, and a minimal amount of swelling are present. Point tenderness is located in the posterior arch just anterior to the calcaneous.

TECHNIQUE:

With the patient lying on the affected side, press with one fingertip on the sole of the foot and mark the most sensitive area with povidone iodine. Refresh your memory of the anatomy with an atlas if necessary, and you'll find that the iodine is over the junction of the conjoined flexor tendon just anterior to its attachment to the calcaneous. Mark the medial border of the foot closest to the tender area as the site of cannula insertion. Fill a 5-ml syringe with 10 mg prednisolone and 1 percent lidocaine and use a sharp 1.5-inch 25-gauge cannula for injection. Insert the cannula toward the first iodine mark and inject 1 ml anaesthetic suspension. If sharp pain is felt, the area of inflammation has been reached. Move the point of the cannula by partly withdrawing it and redirecting the steroid injection distally, transversely, and proximally until total anaesthesia has been accomplished. Be sure to advise the patient that pain will return when the anaesthesia wears off, but also tell the patient that the full effect of the corticosteroid will take forty-eight hours. Pain medication, soft rubber heels, and avoidance of prolonged standing are also advised. (See Fig. 2.)

Second Visit: Repeat the treatment in one week if insufficient relief from pain has been obtained. A third treatment in two weeks is sometimes needed.

Effectiveness: Failures are rare. Marked obesity responds slowly but surely.

Periostitis of the Os Calcis

(Stoned Heel)

INJURY:

Bruising of the periosteum by landing hard on the heel causing inflammation.

SIGNS:

Pain on the heel of the foot owing to inflammation of the periosteum is felt when walking on the heels.

TECHNIQUE:

Have the patient supine with external rotation of the extremity. Press carefully to locate the site of maximum pain and mark with povidone iodine. Do not inject directly through the plantar surface. Use a 5-ml luer-lock syringe filled with 10 mg prednisolone and 1 percent lidocaine. Fit to it a sharp 1.5-inch 25-gauge cannula and insert the point in the medial side of the heel 2 cm proximal to the skin surface in line with the pain area. Slowly inject as you insert the cannula until the patient indicates that the inflamed area has been reached. Inject the entire area by multiple puncture to layer the prednisolone throughout the affected area. A sponge heel insert may afford additional relief.

Second Visit: A week later, repeat the treatment if needed.

Effectiveness: Usually two treatments are adequate. If the patient is excessively overweight, more injections will be necessary and walking on cement pavements should be limited.

Synovitis Ankle Joint

INJURY:

Sprain, intra-articular fracture, crush injury, and gout can cause inflammation of the lining synovia of the ankle joint.

SIGNS:

Pain on weight-bearing dorsiflexion is usually present with or without an obvious accompanying injury.

TECHNIQUE:

With the patient supine and a small bolster beneath the knee, identify the anterior margin of the tibia and mark the point where the medial joint space is located. Half fill a 10-ml luer-lock syringe with 1 percent lidocaine and apply a sharp 1.5-inch 22-gauge cannula to it. Feel the anterior tibial tendon and move it laterally one cm. Enter the joint slowly by injecting lidocaine ahead of the cannula until you are well into the superior space between the tibia and the talus along the medial border. Be sure to stay medial to the anterior tibial artery. Inject the remaining lidocaine and aspirate as much joint fluid as possible. Remove the syringe, leaving the cannula in place, and fill a fresh syringe with 10 mg prednisolone in 5 ml 1 percent lidocaine. Inject the joint through the same cannula and remove it. Have the patient obtain maximum motion before applying an ace bandage or a plastic splint. If the joint fluid is bloody, irrigate with 10 ml lidocaine, but do not inject prednisolone. (See Fig. 3.)

Second Visit: In one week, a second aspiration can be done on a joint that was filled with blood and prednisolone can be injected. Those joints that were free from blood can be given a second injection of prednisolone in 4 percent dextrose in lidocaine if pain and swelling continue.

Effectiveness: Rarely is it necessary to see the patient more than twice, unless a fracture, arthritis, or gout is producing symptoms.

Outer-Ankle Sprain

(Stress Injuries of Lateral Ankle Ligaments)

INJURY:

Partial tear of the anterior talofibular ligament is the most frequent injury. Next in frequency and occurring along with the talofibular are tears of the superior peroneal retinaculum and the deeper-lying calcaneofibular ligament.

SIGNS:

Pain, hemorrhagic discoloration, swelling, and inability to bear weight are present. Very marked instability occurs in complete ruptures of the major ligaments.

TECHNIQUE:

With the patient supine on the examining table and a soft bolster beneath the knee, prepare the skin with povidone-iodine soap and surgical solution. Fill a 5-ml syringe with 10 mg prednisolone and 1 percent lidocaine and inject the swollen subcutaneous tissues at 1-inch intervals using a sharp ⅝-inch cannula. Limit the increments to units of 1 ml. Mark the tibio-talar joint horizontally with povidone iodine and draw a vertical line over the tendon of the tibialis anterior as it crosses the joint. Half fill a 10-ml luer-lock syringe with 1 percent lidocaine and fit it with a sharp 22-gauge 1.5-inch cannula. Push the tendon toward the midline of the tibia and inject 0.5 ml lidocaine into the subcutaneous tissue just above the joint. Penetrate the joint and aspirate to determine the presence of blood. Inject the lidocaine and aspirate repeatedly to remove all blood. Leave the cannula in place and remove the syringe with sterile technique and refill it with fresh lidocaine if more irrigation is necessary. Finally, inject the joint with 10 mg prednisolone in 3 ml 1 percent lidocaine to relieve pain and swelling from inflammation. Apply a snug, but not tight, elastic bandage from the base of the toes to just above the ankle. Instruct the patient to elevate the ankle and exercise the toes and move the ankle to reduce swelling, and to use the elastic bandage while ambulatory. (See Fig. 4.)

Second Visit: One week later, most of the swelling will be gone and the ligament injury can be identified. Fingertip pressure will locate the damaged ligaments. Fill a 2-ml syringe with 8 percent dextrose in 1 percent lidocaine and use a sharp ⅝-inch 25-gauge cannula for treatment at the ligament-bone junction with 0.2-ml increments of solution. Instruct the patient to avoid stressing the ankle ligaments.

Effectiveness: Complete relief of symptoms may require three or four treatments, a week apart. Six weeks from the last injection, most patients are able to return to full activity. Some individuals will need a sugar-tong type of plaster of Paris ankle support to prevent inversion during the treatment period. This cast is easily applied with an elastic bandage and can be removed for bathing and at bedtime. Complete ligament rupture with marked ankle instability will need surgical repair.

Inner-Ankle Sprain

(Deltoid Ligament Sprain)

INJURY:

Partial tears of the medial ankle ligaments (deltoid) can occur at the tibia, the navicular, the talus, and the calcaneus.

SIGNS:

Pain, tenderness, and swelling on the medial side of the ankle joint must be investigated for the nature and extent of injury.

TECHNIQUE:

Initial treatment is directed toward reduction of acute pain, inflammation, and swelling.

With the patient supine and the lower extremity externally rotated, inject the areas of pain and swelling with 1 percent lidocaine containing 1 mg prednisolone per ml until no tenderness is present. Apply an elastic bandage if the patient is able to bear weight. Use a removable, molded plaster, sugar-tong cast if pain is too severe to permit walking. Instruct the patient to remove the dressing when in bed and to elevate the foot half the waking hours during the first week. Arch support should be worn constantly to prevent any pronation of the foot.

Second Visit: After one week, identify the injured ligaments and inject them with 0.2-ml increments of 8 percent dextrose at the periosteal attachments to bone. Do not inject more than is necessary to obtain anaesthesia. Reapply the cast if the ankle was too painful for an elastic bandage on the first visit. Caution the patient that relief from pain does not mean complete healing.

Effectiveness: At least four ligament injections will be needed in those ankles requiring a cast. From two to four injections will promote healing in stable ankles, and complete healing should be present within six weeks of the last injection.

Achilles Tendinitis

INJURY:
Inflammation of the tendon sheath can occur from repetitive jumping, running, and sudden stretching.

SIGNS:
Pain and tenderness along the Achilles tendon. Pain on rising on the balls of the feet. Swelling is present in fiber ruptures.

TECHNIQUE:
With the patient prone and a bolster beneath the anterior ankles, use a fingertip to locate the tender areas. Compress the tendon between thumb and index finger to locate small areas of swelling where some of the tendon fibers are stressed or torn. Inject the tendon sheath in all the tender areas with 1 percent lidocaine containing 1 mg prednisolone per ml, using a 25-gauge cannula until no tenderness remains. Test for partial ruptures of the tendon fibers by compression and inject 0.1 ml 8.0 percent dextrose in lidocaine at intervals of 5 mm into the areas of tenderness until they are pain free. Medial, lateral, and posterior surfaces of the tendon are easily injected. The anterior surface, which is often affected, is more difficult. Caution the patient to avoid stressing the tendon. Instruct the patient to lift the foot when walking instead of rising on the toes and striding.

Second Visit: In one or two weeks, depending on the response to initial treatment, evaluate the nature of disability by differentiating between the pain within the tendon and that in the tendon sheath. Treat as on the initial visit.

Effectiveness: Many patients improve significantly within two or three visits, but many do not respond well to treatment. Six weeks of nonstress of the tendon is necessary for complete healing and some individuals are not able to accept this. A moderate heel elevation on the injured side will remind the patient to avoid rising on the toes when walking.

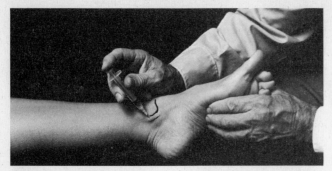

Fig. 1

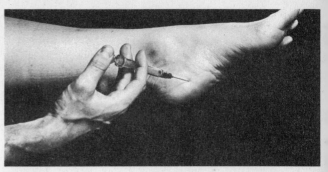

Fig. 2

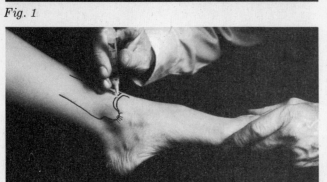

Fig. 3

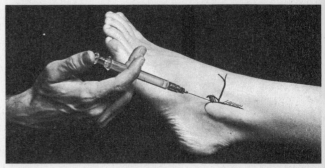

Fig. 4

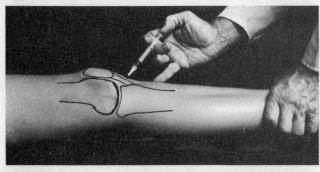

Fig. 5

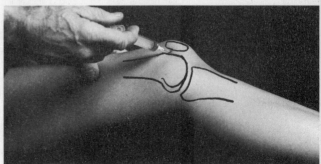

Fig. 6

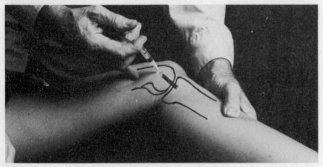

Fig. 7

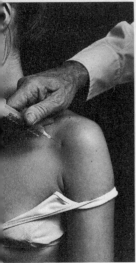

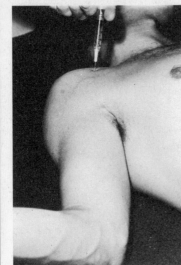

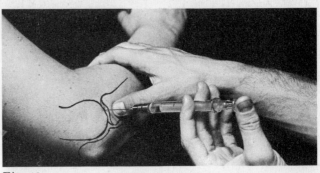

Fig. 12

Fig. 8

Fig. 9

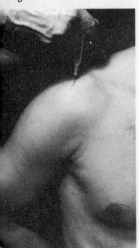

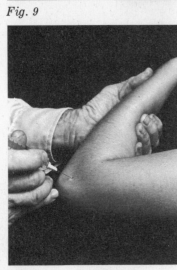

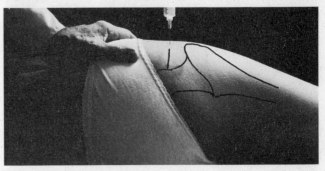

Fig. 13

Fig. 10

Fig. 11

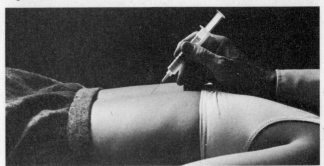

Fig. 14

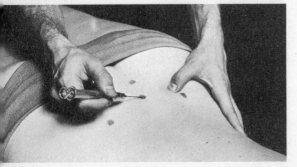

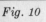

Fig. 15

The Knee

Patella Ligament Strain

(Patella Tendinitis)

INJURY:

Jumping and running stress the patella ligament in its substance and especially at the attachment to the lower pole of the patella. Tiny avulsions occur at the periosteal junction.

SIGNS:

Pain at the lower pole of the patella or in the tendon substance occurs on resisted extension of the knee. Climbing stairs is usually painful.

TECHNIQUE:

With the patient supine and the knee flexed only to 90°, mark the lower pole of the patella where maximum tenderness is present. Inject the ligament bone junction with 0.2 ml increments of 8 percent dextrose in 1 percent lidocaine using a sharp 25-gauge cannula. Test by resisted extension as well as by pressure. Ligament injuries can be injected in the same way in the substance of the ligament at the point of maximum compression tenderness. Test after injection. Caution against jumping.

Second Visit: Repeat the treatment if symptoms are still present.

Effectiveness: No failures are present in my small group. Up to four injections using minimal amounts at one-week intervals are sometimes required.

Suprapatellar Tendinitis

INJURY:
Contusion or extreme stress will cause tendon and periosteal inflammation at the superior pole and lateral margins of the patella where tiny avulsions occur.

SIGNS:
Pain and tenderness at the upper pole of the patella medial and/or lateral on resisted knee extension are the major signs.

TECHNIQUE:
With the patient supine and the affected knee fully flexed, identify the tender areas on the upper pole and mark with povidone iodine. Fill a 5 ml luer-lock syringe with 8 percent dextrose in 1 percent lidocaine and fit it with a 1.5-inch 25-gauge sharp cannula. Hold the knee firmly with one hand and slowly insert the cannula through the skin at the points of tenderness, injecting the local anaesthetic ahead of the point. Aim at the tendon insertion and inject 0.2 ml. Sharp stinging pain occurs only at the point of inflammation. Slowly inject 0.2-ml increments of dextrose lidocaine until anaesthesia is complete. Test for ability to extend the knee against resistance. Caution against kicking, jumping, or running during the four-week recovery phase.
　Second Visit: Repeat the injection of dextrose lidocaine in one week.
　Effectiveness: Usually three injections effect a "cure." Since the dextrose is a stimulus for repair, a full four weeks of diminished activity is necessary for complete healing after the last injection.

Infrapatellar Bursitis

INJURY:
Inflammation of the deep infrapatellar bursae beneath the ligament, between the patella and the tibial tubercle, can occur frequently.

SIGNS:
Full knee flexion is sometimes painful and local tenderness is present beneath the ligament. Firm thumb pressure causes pain, as does kneeling with full weight on the injured knee.

TECHNIQUE:
With the patient supine on the examining table, locate the exact area of pain with the fingertip and mark it with povidone iodine. Knee extended with muscles relaxed permits easy injection of the deep bursa. Use a luer-lock syringe and a sharp 1.5-inch 25-gauge needle to inject 1 percent lidocaine with 1 mg prednisolone per ml. Fill the bursa with 3 to 5 ml, then have the patient completely flex and extend the knee to distribute the suspension. Total

relief from tenderness and pain must be obtained. Caution against kneeling for four to six weeks. (See Fig. 5.)

Second Visit: Repeat the treatment of the first visit if pain returns.

Effectiveness: A maximum of two treatments is usually enough to obtain full relief.

Traumatic Inflammation of the Knee Joint

INJURY:

Inflammation of synovial lining with or without fluid formation is often due to both internal and external irritation by arthritis, loose bony bodies in the joint, a fall landing on the knee, a collision in sports, or an accident in a car. Gout or pseudo-gout cause formation of crystals which will also irritate and inflame synovia.

SIGNS:

Pain, local heat, swelling, tenderness, loss of motion, and impaired weight bearing may be present in varying degrees. Flexion is always more limited than extension. Swelling of the knee joint will frequently occur as a secondary phenomenon with most knee ligament injuries. In these cases, unless the cause is treated simultaneously with the joint inflammation, joint swelling will return.

TECHNIQUE:

Patient lying supine with, at times, a small bolster beneath the knee is the easiest position. Locate the patella and mark the skin with povidone iodine along the medial inferior margin. If fluid is present, aspirate this before injection with a sharp 1.5-inch 22-gauge cannula. With one finger, gently push the patella laterally and inject 5 ml 1 percent lidocaine through the skin into the space beneath the patella. After two minutes, aspirate the joint fluid completely. Disengage the syringe from the cannula and empty the contents into a sterile tube for later microscopic examination. Using a fresh syringe containing 20 mg prednisolone in 8 ml lidocaine, attach it to the 22-gauge cannula that remains in place under the patella, and inject the contents into the joint space. Remove the syringe with attached cannula and obtain maximum range of knee-joint motion to disperse the suspension of prednisolone. If no joint aspiration is to be done, use a 1.5-inch gauge cannula to inject the joint with 8 ml lidocaine, 20 mg prednisolone mixture. (See Fig. 6.)

Second Visit: One, or at the most two, injections may be given one or two weeks apart. If the synovitis continues, ligament or meniscus injury should be investigated more thoroughly.

Effectiveness: Simple transient injuries producing synovitis are relieved with a single injection. Osteoarthritic joint changes can be relieved for as long as three months by injecting 20 mg prednisolone in 8 ml 8 percent dextrose in lidocaine.

Lateral Collateral Ligament

INJURY:
Partial ligament rupture or avulsion from bone.

SIGNS:
Pain on varus stress.

TECHNIQUE:
With the patient lying on the unaffected side, mark the skin over each positive area with povidone iodine. For injuries to ligaments and attachments, use a 3-ml luer-lock syringe and a sharp 1.5-inch 25-gauge cannula. Inject 8 percent dextrose in 1 percent lidocaine into the positive areas with 0.2-ml amounts in adjacent areas until total anaesthesia is present.

Second Visit: Seven to ten days after the initial injections, repeat the treatment in all tender areas. Decide on further treatment depending upon the amount of local reaction to dextrose lidocaine or to corticosteroid.

Effectiveness: Ligament injuries at the periosteal junction will heal in three treatments at seven-to-ten-day intervals. One to three visits will improve most injuries demonstrating tendinitis.

Medial Collateral Ligament Area

INJURY:
1. Partial ligament tear.
2. Complete ligament tear.
3. Partial ligament avulsion from bone.
4. Complete ligament avulsion from bone.
5. Adhesions between ligament and subjacent tissues.
6. Bursitis beneath the ligament.

SIGNS:
1. Partial tear causes pain on valgus stress and local tenderness.
2. Complete tear results in marked instability.
3. Adhesions limit motion, cause pain and tenderness.
4. Bursitis permits full motion with local pain and tenderness.

TECHNIQUE (LIGAMENT INJURIES):
Localize the exact point of tenderness with a fingertip and apply a 1 cm dot of povidone iodine to the skin. Fill a 3-ml luer-lock syringe with 8 percent dextrose in 1 percent lidocaine and equip it with a sharp 25-gauge 1.5-inch cannula. Hold the skin firmly in place with a fingertip and insert the point through the iodine down to the level of injury. The

patient will describe a sudden acute pain when the area of inflammation is reached. Inject slowly 0.2- or 0.3-ml solution and wait until pain is relieved before withdrawing the point to the subcutaneous level and reinserting it to an adjacent area of inflammation. Inject 0.2 ml every 4 mm until the injured tissue is totally anaesthetic. Periosteal attachments and ligaments will heal more rapidly after injection. (See Fig. 7.) Complete tear is a surgical emergency.

TECHNIQUE (ADHESIONS):

Have the patient flex the knee until motion is stopped by pain. Dot the skin with povidone iodine over the point of maximum pain and inject beneath the ligament with 3 ml 1 percent lidocaine containing 10 mg of prednisolone. Slowly extend and flex the knee to increase the range of motion. If flexion is not yet full range, inject a second 3 ml of prednisolone suspension in lidocaine. Instruct the patient in active assisted exercises.

TECHNIQUE (BURSITIS):

With the knee flexed to 90°, palpate the joint line anteromedially with a fingertip moving posteriorly until an area of maximum pain is found. Mark with povidone iodine and inject, using the same technique as in the treatment of adhesions. Have the patient limit physical activity to permit the bursitis to subside. After forty-eight to seventy-two hours, the patient may resume full activity.

Second Visit: Repeat treatment in those patients who have reached maximum benefit one week after the initial visit. Most will have pain after the lidocaine has lost its effect and they will complain that they were temporarily worse. Two or three visits are enough to treat adequately 90 percent of patients with medial collateral ligament injuries described in this section. For complete healing to take place, six to eight weeks of protected activity must be observed for partial ligament tears.

Effectiveness: Injection promotes rapid healing in partial ligament tears. A few patients will obtain years of complete relief from pain after one treatment visit. Three or four injections, a week apart, will "cure" more than 90 percent of the remaining group. Bursitis usually improves with a maximum of three injections a week apart. Limitation of motion, which is due to adhesions, may require considerable active assisted exercise and two or three weeks between treatment visits.

Medial Coronary Ligament

INJURY:

A tearing of the coronary ligament of the medial meniscus away from its attachment to the tibia just below the anterior and anteromedial border of the medial tibial plateau. This can occur at the periosteal attachment or the portion just proximal to the periosteum.

SIGNS:

Local pain is made much more intense by twisting the knee while weight bearing or by passive external rotation of the leg. Marked tenderness is present along the anteromedial border of the medial tibial plateau.

TECHNIQUE:

With the patient supine, flex the knee to 90° and mark the area of tenderness with povidone iodine. Fill a 3-ml luer-lock syringe with 8 percent dextrose in 1 percent lidocaine and inject into the periosteum and ligament with a sharp 1.5-inch 25-gauge cannula. Use only enough solution to obtain total anaesthesia. Warn the patient to avoid weight-bearing twisting motion and running. No pain-producing activity is permitted.

Second Visit: Repeat the treatment if pain or tenderness is present. Continue the patient on reduced activity but encourage nonweight-bearing flexion extension and quadriceps-setting exercise.

Effectiveness: Rapid healing is obtained with a minimum of two and a maximum of six treatment visits. Return to full use is not possible until six weeks after the last treatment. Recent expert opinion indicates that repair of the coronary ligament is much to be preferred over the practice of removing the meniscus on the injured side. Open operation and suture of the torn ligament is advised.

The Shoulder

Acute Subdeltoid Bursitis

INJURY:

Inflammation of the subdeltoid bursa can result from a single injury, such as a fall on the outstretched hand, or from repetitive motion, such as window washing. It is more likely to occur in older people, whose production of cortisone by the suprarenal glands is less efficient.

SIGNS:

Pain and swelling will be present in proportion to the degree of inflammation. Loss of motion is usually complete. The affected shoulder may be warm to touch. Passive abduction is extremely limited and painful. Passive external rotation is also limited and painful, but less so. Passive internal rotation is slightly limited and painful.

TECHNIQUE:

Have the patient sit upright with elbow flexed and the forearm lying in the least painful position. Dot the skin over the head of the humerus with povidone iodine at intervals of 3 cm in the places of maximum tenderness and inject the bursa with 10 ml 1 percent lidocaine containing 20 mg prednisolone. Use a luer-lock syringe fitted with a sharp 1.5-inch 25-gauge cannula and make several punctures of the bursa through a single skin puncture by withdrawing the point of the cannula to the subcutaneous level and reinserting it at an

308

angle before continuing the injection. When anaesthesia permits, slowly rotate the humerus with the point in the partially withdrawn position and inject the total bursa. If 10 mg steroid suspension is not enough, fill the syringe with 10 mg prednisolone in 5 ml lidocaine and treat remaining areas until a full range of rotation and elevation can be obtained. (See Fig. 8.)

Second Visit: Encourage the patient to return for a second treatment within one week to ensure that a full range of painless motion will be retained. During this visit it should be possible to inject multiple areas of the bursa by rotating the humerus and by pressure testing for residual areas of tenderness.

Effectiveness: A first attack of bursitis responds readily if it is treated within forty-eight hours. After that time the surfaces of the bursa begin to form adhesions with progressive loss of motion. More than two treatment visits will be needed, but the prognosis for "cure" is excellent.

Chronic Subdeltoid Bursitis

INJURY:
Repeated attacks of subacute bursitis will result in the formation of considerable granulation tissue, producing a nodular surface in the subdeltoid bursa. Some pockets of synovitis enclosed by adhesions will be present.

SIGNS:
Low-grade recurrent episodes of pain occur at certain points in the range of shoulder motion. Although more than 70 percent to 95 percent of normal motion is present in most patients, some will demonstrate marked restriction of the range. Loss of some external and internal rotation and loss of 25 percent of elevation can be accompanied by crepitus and pain. Local tenderness is definite but not acute. A painful arc of motion is often a consistent sign.

TECHNIQUE:
With the patient sitting in a chair, determine the range of rotation and elevation. Note the areas of subjective pain and objective tenderness at the end of the ranges of motion. Mark these areas with povidone iodine. (See illustration for acute bursitis, page 157.) Fill a luerlock syringe as in the treatment of acute subdeltoid bursitis and obtain maximum motion by injecting units of 3 ml 1 percent lidocaine via the marked areas. Maintain some rotation while injecting, but do not stress the deltoid too much. Separate adhesions by filling up the bursa completely. This takes a minimum of 30 cc of 0.5 percent lidocaine. After reaching the maximum range of motion, inject the 0.5 percent lidocaine containing 20 mg of prednisolone. Manipulate the shoulder to distribute the suspended corticosteroid throughout the bursa.

Second Visit: One or two weeks after the initial injection and manipulation, repeat the procedure if needed.

Effectiveness: Most patients will improve with two to four injections if they can cooperate in the program of pendulum and active assisted elevation and rotation exercises.

Subscapularis Tendinitis

INJURY:
Inflammation of the subscapularis tendon in the area of attachment to the lesser tuberosity of the humerus is one of the most common shoulder injuries.

SIGNS:
Pain is produced high up on the lesser tuberosity at the junction of the head and neck of the humerus with strong adduction of the arm, which is adducted to 90°. Resisted medial rotation is painful. Passive lateral rotation is often painful as well. Local tenderness is present just medial to the bicipital groove of the humerus shoulder. Pain on overhand serve in tennis and on throwing a ball is also diagnostic.

TECHNIQUE:
With the patient in supine position, identify the long head of the biceps in the bicipital groove. Externally rotate the arm and mark the tender attachment of the subscapularis muscle with povidone iodine. Fill a luer-lock syringe with 10 mg prednisolone in 5 ml 1 percent lidocaine containing 4 percent dextrose and fit it with a sharp 1.5-inch 25-gauge cannula. With the patient maintaining an externally rotated humerus, gently inject at right angles to the skin to cover the tendon area with the prednisolone suspension. Probe with the point of the cannula to locate areas of inflammation and treat until no tenderness and no injection pain are present. (See Fig. 9.)

Second Visit: Repeat the initial treatment in seven to ten days if only partial improvement is present.

Effectiveness: When only the subscapularis is involved, considerable relief from pain is evident after the first visit. A full four to six weeks of nonstressful activity is necessary to permit complete healing. Significant stimulus to repair is provided by 8 percent dextrose in lidocaine after the initial inflammation has improved. Symptoms will govern the duration of treatment.

Supraspinatus Tendinitis and Tendon Rupture

INJURY:
Repeated friction of the tendon on the undersurface of the edge of the acromion will cause inflammation. Sometimes a calcific deposit acts like a foreign body and produces a severe inflammatory response when it becomes large enough. Sudden strong pressure against the partially elevated arm can rupture the tendon. This usually occurs in older individuals.

Constant pain, or pain on motion. Pain can be referred all the way to the wrist. Resisted adduction is painful. (Note: If pain is felt on release of resisted motion, subscapularis or infraspinatus is at fault.)

TECHNIQUE:
With the patient sitting, hand behind the back resting on the chair seat, internal rotation of the humerus will bring the supraspinatus tendon anterior to the acromion. Identify the painful tendon with a fingertip and mark the skin with povidone iodine. Fill a 5-ml syringe with 10 mg prednisolone and 1 percent lidocaine and use a sharp 1.5-inch 25-gauge cannula for injection. Insert the point through the skin down to the tendon and inject 1 ml suspension over the surface. Probe with the cannula to determine if the tendon is resilient and tough or is abnormal in offering no resistance to the penetrating point. A gap in the continuity of the tissue will indicate a tendon tear. If the tendon is normal, inject the remaining steroid suspension over the surface.

Symptomatic calcific tendinitis may be treated by injecting the calcium to disperse it. Calcific deposits can vary in density from a semiliquid mass contained within the paratenon to a dense, hard, bonelike mass that protrudes from the tendon into the subdeltoid bursa. Injecting directly into the semiliquid mass will rupture the encompassing membrane and disperse the calcium. A sharp 22-gauge cannula will be needed to break up the dense calcific deposits.

Healing of abnormally soft tendon can be stimulated by local injection of 0.1-ml increments of 8 percent dextrose in lidocaine. Advise the patient that surgical repair may be needed if injection is not successful. (See Fig. 10.)

Second Visit: Repeat the initial treatment in one week if pain is still present. Calcium dispersion can be monitored by X-ray examination. Test abnormal tendons by the same technique as was used on the first visit and repeat the local injection of 0.1-ml increments of 8 percent dextrose in lidocaine. Warn the patient against forceful use of the shoulder for a period of two weeks after treatment of inflammation. In tendon injuries, this is especially important.

Effectiveness: Superficial tendinitis will respond to one or two treatments with corticosteroid. Calcific deposits that are proved to be dispersed by X-ray examination rarely need more than three visits. Partial tears of the tendon will require four to six injections at one- or two-week intervals. A partial tendon tear will need an additional six-week period of healing after the last dextrose injection.

Infraspinatus Tendinitis

INJURY:
Partial tear of the tendon at its insertion posterior to the supraspinatus tendon is a common injury. Inflammation may also be present in the body of the tendon.

SIGNS:

Pain, low grade, is present with acute pain on playing a backhand in tennis or on reaching behind with arm externally rotated. Resisted external rotation usually reproduces the pain. Testing should be done at different degrees of rotation.

TECHNIQUE:

Have the patient lying on the uninjured side and place the injured arm behind the back to produce fixed internal rotation of the humerus. Fill a 10-ml luer-lock syringe with 20 mg prednisolone in 1 percent lidocaine and apply a sharp 1.5-inch 25-gauge cannula. Mark the area of maximum tenderness with povidone iodine and inject the surface over the tendon with 3 ml suspension. Withdraw the point and redirect it at an angle to cover the entire tendon area and complete the injection to abolish inflammation. No strong use of the muscle is permitted until the next examination.

Second Visit: One week after the initial treatment, inject the tendon only at the point of pain with small 0.1-ml increments of 8 percent dextrose in lidocaine to stimulate repair.

Effectiveness: Usually a maximum of three or four treatments will be needed along with a four- to six-week period of light activity.

Biceps Tendinitis

INJURY:

Usually inflammation of the long head of the biceps muscle takes place as it enters the bicipital groove in the head of the humerus. This long tendon is subject to rubbing in its long course into the shoulder joint, and inflammation can occur at any point from high on the humerus to inside the joint.

SIGNS:

Pain occurs near the anterior shoulder or the upper arm when the biceps muscle is strongly contracted in resisted flexion. Tenderness along the tendon is also present.

TECHNIQUE:

With the patient sitting or supine, mark the point of maximum tenderness with povidone iodine and fill a 5-ml luer-lock syringe with 10 mg prednisolone in 1 percent lidocaine. Apply a sharp 1.5-inch 25-gauge cannula and inject the tendon sheath of the biceps. Use a fingertip lightly pressed along the tendon below the bicipital groove to feel the fluid distending the sheath of the biceps tendon and complete the injection to cover the entire tendon surface. After three minutes, test for pain-free motion to be sure that treatment is complete.

Second Visit: Repeat the treatment in one week, then at two-week intervals if necessary.

Effectiveness: Usually three treatments are enough. I cannot recall any patients whose symptoms continued beyond the third visit.

The Elbow

Tennis Elbow

INJURY:

Inflammation or tear of the extensor carpi radialis brevis at the teno-periosteal junction is the most frequent cause of the so-called tennis elbow. The tendon of the brachioradialis and conjoined extensor tendons of the forearm glide across a bursa overlying the lateral epicondyle of the humerus. Sufficient friction here will also produce a severe inflammation of the bursa, which may be mistaken for tendinitis. Some patients have, in addition, a tendinitis with areas of necrosis involving the substance of the tendon.

SIGNS:

Local pain, tenderness, and inability to dorsiflex the wrist against resistance may be very marked.

TECHNIQUE:

Supine or sitting positions are satisfactory. Pure bursitis is best treated by local injection with prednisolone in lidocaine. Fill a 5-ml luer-lock syringe with 10 mg prednisolone in 1 percent lidocaine and fit to it a sharp 1.5-inch 25-gauge cannula. Mark the point of maximum pain with povidone iodine and inject after penetrating the overlying tendon with a single motion down to the bursa overlying the bone. Use 1 ml medication and test for resisted dorsiflexion after two minutes. If tendon tenderness and disability are still present, inject the tendon by stippling with 0.1 ml prednisolone using the minimal amount to obtain complete pain-free function. (See Fig. 11.)

Second Visit: Repeat the injection in one or two weeks if disability continues. Alternate 8 percent dextrose in lidocaine with decreasing amounts of prednisolone in patients with tendinitis.

Effectiveness: Half the patients will be "cured" in one or two visits. Three or four treatment visits should be adequate for the other half. If pain persists, surgical treatment should be considered.

Golfer's Elbow

(Tendinitis of the Common Flexor Tendon of the Elbow; Medial Epiconylar Bursitis)

INJURY:

Inflammation of the conjoined tendon of the flexor muscles of the forearm along the medial condyle of the humerus is the cause of disability from excessive use. Often there is a bursa on the medial epicondyle of the humerus, which becomes inflamed and cannot, at first, be differentiated from a tendinitis.

SIGNS:

Local pain over the medial condyle of the humerus is associated with loss of ability to volar flex the hand at the wrist against resistance. Any attempt to tighten the grip when shaking hands may also cause pain on the medial side of the elbow.

TECHNIQUE:

Have the patient sit facing the examining table or supine upon it. With the elbow flexed to 90° and the arm resting on the table surface, identify and mark the area of maximum tenderness. If the conjoined flexor tendon is very sensitive to pressure for several centimeters, mark it accordingly with povidone iodine. Fill a 3-ml luer-lock syringe with 5 mg prednisolone in 4 percent dextrose, 1 percent lidocaine, and apply a sharp 1.5-inch 25-gauge cannula. Test for an epicondyle bursitis by injecting the tip of the epicondyle with 0.2 ml suspension and after two minutes test the flexor power of the wrist. If no significant relief has been obtained, inject the tendon by multiple 0.1-ml increments until no tenderness and no pain are present. Avoid piercing the ulnar nerve by placing one finger along the posterior aspect of the epicondyle and keep the injection anterior and slightly lateral.

Second Visit: If necessary, treat a second time one or two weeks after the first with elimination of the prednisolone using 8 percent dextrose in 1 percent lidocaine to stipple the tendon.

Effectiveness: Very few patients need more than two visits.

Traumatic Arthritis of the Elbow Joint

INJURY:

Loss of smooth articular surface in any part of the joint will erode the apposing cartilage. Fragments broken off into the joint will irregularly destroy cartilage and later injure the synovia to produce a synovitis.

SIGNS:

Swelling, pain, and limitation of motion are present in varying degrees. Flexion is more limited than extension.

TECHNIQUE:

The patient may be sitting or supine depending on the extent of pain and disability. Accurately measure the range of motion and record this as a baseline for efficacy of treatment. Mark the lateral skin area with povidone iodine directly over the junction of the head of the radius, the ulna, and the capitulum. Fill a 5-ml luer-lock syringe with 10 mg prednisolone in 8 percent dextrose 1 percent lidocaine solution. Fit a sharp 1.5-inch 25-gauge cannula to the syringe and insert it through the skin in the triangle formed by the radial head, the ulna, and the capitulum. It helps to place a forefinger on the lateral elbow joint and rotate the head of the radius for exact location. Flex the elbow to 100° to provide space for the cannula and inject. (See Fig. 12.)

Second Visit: After one or two weeks, measure the range of elbow motion and repeat the treatment if some increase in motion is present.

Effectiveness: Remarkable improvement in motion, swelling, and pain follow three or four injections at two-week intervals in some patients. If improvement stops, and symptoms do not permit adequate function, arrange for the patient to consult an operating orthopedist regarding the necessity for surgery.

Triceps Tendon Strain

INJURY:

Partial tears of the triceps tendon resulting from overstressing are frequent among weight lifters. Inflammation can occur with repetitive motion causing rubbing or can be due to a direct blow from a hard object and/or the bursa over the back of the joint capsule can become inflamed.

SIGNS:

Resisted extension where the muscle contracts isometrically will cause pain in partial tears. Doing a military press with a barbell will produce pain in a tendinitis. Pain is always directly in the injured tendon.

TECHNIQUE:

Have the patient sit with the arm behind the axillary line with the volar aspect of the flexed elbow resting on the back of the chair. Mark the area of maximum tenderness with povidone iodine and fill a 5-ml syringe with 4 percent dextrose in 1 percent lidocaine. Fit it with a sharp 1.5-inch 25-gauge cannula and inject both superficial and deep to the tendon, using at least 1.5 ml anaesthetic suspension at each level. Wait three minutes and test for complete freedom from pain. Repeat injection until all pain is gone. Inflamed bursae can be treated by local injection of a prednisolone suspension.

Second Visit: Partial tears will need 4 percent dextrose in 1 percent lidocaine. Use a sharp ⅝-inch cannula and inject the tendon by multiple puncture with 0.2-ml increments of solution until total pain relief is accomplished. Within one or two weeks, repeat the treatment if necessary.

Effectiveness: I have had better results with noncompetitive athletes than with weight lifters in competition. Very light workouts may be done for four to six weeks during the healing period.

The Hip and Thigh

Synovitis of the Hip Joint

INJURY:

Bruising of the lining of the hip joint during violent activity, or just running, will result in marked local inflammation. In older patients, osteoarthritis plus unusual activity will injure the synovia of the hip joint.

SIGNS:

Groin pain and tenderness with a marked limping gait are initial signs. Examination demonstrates severe pain on internal rotation of the hip at 90° flexion and also in extension.

TECHNIQUE:

Have the patient lie on the good side with the good hip and knee flexed. The affected hip should be in extension with the knee straight to permit introduction of a sharp cannula into the lateral side of the hip joint. Mark the top of the greater trochanter with povidone iodine and place a second spot on the skin one inch proximal to the trochanter. Use a 10-ml luer-lock syringe and a 3½-inch sharp 19-gauge cannula. Fill with 20 mg prednisolone in 1 percent lidocaine and inject the joint by pointing directly medially with the hip in a little internal rotation. Try to test your direction by following the neck of the femur up into the joint capsule. Use only 7 ml in the joint to avoid intra-articular pressure. Caution the patient to rest for twenty-four hours and slowly increase activity to normal after three days. (See Fig. 13.)

Second Visit: Only half of my patients obtained a "cure" with one treatment. Ninety percent of the rest needed a second injection.

Effectiveness: Simple traumatic synovial injuries are easily treated by injection of prednisolone. Osteoarthritis causing synovitis of the hip joint will need an injection every three months.

Rectus Femoris Tendinitis, or Muscle Tear

INJURY:
Stressing the rectus femoris muscle or tendons beyond the elastic point will cause tendon inflammation or muscle tear.

SIGNS:
Local tenderness and pain on hip flexion from 180° extension is present over the two tendons of origin of the rectus femoris distally in the muscle tissue of both areas.

TECHNIQUE:
With the patient supine, identify and mark the point of maximum tenderness with povidone iodine. Palpate the femoral artery and avoid it by keeping all injections lateral to avoid the nerve when injecting the areas of the muscle or tendon. Fill a 10-ml luer-lock syringe with 10 mg prednisolone in 1 percent lidocaine and apply a sharp 1.5-inch 25-gauge cannula depending on the depth to the injured tissue. Enter the skin perpendicularly and slowly penetrate to the level of inflammation while injecting the anaesthetic mixture. When the patient complains of a sudden burning pain, stop penetration and slowly infiltrate that area with several ml prednisolone in lidocaine until pain is relieved. After three minutes, have the patient stand and flex the hip with the knee straight on the injured side. Absence of pain indicates adequate treatment.

Second Visit: Repeat the injection in two weeks if disability continues. Use 8 percent dextrose for the tendons in one- or two-ml amounts by small 0.1-ml increments at five-minute intervals until the pain is gone.

Effectiveness: Tendinitis usually responds within two treatments if inflammation is not too severe. More treatment may be needed in severe cases.

Thigh Muscles, Aspiration of Hematoma

INJURY:
Crush injuries rupture large blood vessels in the thigh muscles, especially the vastus lateralis. Blood has no exit, unless an open wound is present, and forms a hematoma. Often a small arteriole is ruptured with very rapid onset of bleeding, which stops only when the pressure of the hematoma sufficiently compresses the arteriole.

SIGNS:

Local swelling may be unusually great, containing more than a pint of blood. Pain can be very severe because of internal pressure.

TECHNIQUE:

Have the patient supine on the examining table with both lower extremities extended. Prepare the area as necessary with povidone iodine as the final skin treatment and fill a 10-ml or 20-ml luer-lock syringe with 1 percent lidocaine and anaesthetize the skin and subcutaneous tissue directly over the hematoma with 1 percent lidocaine, usually about 3 ml. Remove the fine cannula used for skin injection with a sterile needle holder and substitute a sharp 3.5-inch 18-gauge cannula. Insert this through the skin, injecting more lidocaine as necessary to prevent pain in the deep tissues, and enter the hematoma. Aspirate by partially withdrawing the plunger from the syringe without contaminating the barrel and remove units of 10 ml or more depending upon the size of the syringe. If clots tend to block the cannula, fill a fresh syringe with 1 percent lidocaine or sterile saline and dilute the contents of the hematoma. Observe sterile technique and remove the entire hematoma if possible by emptying and replacing the aspiration syringe. If clotting prevents adequate aspiration, leave 10-ml 1 percent lidocaine within the hematoma and repeat the procedure in twenty-four hours. Prescribe a broad-spectrum antibiotic if a second aspiration will be done within twenty-four hours and apply a firm, but not tight, elastic bandage from foot to just above the hematoma.

Second Visit: If all the blood has been removed, a second visit can be delayed for one week. At that time, judge the necessity for further aspiration and caution the patient to avoid sports activities until no tenderness, swelling, or pain has been present for three weeks.

Effectiveness: Usually a single-treatment visit is adequate because almost all patients have been waiting for a week or more before coming to the doctor. The hematoma is liquid, easily aspirated, and easily irrigated clean. The absence of residual blood avoids a return of fluid by osmotic pressure.

Trochanteric Bursitis

(Greater Trochanter)

INJURY:

Inflammation can result from repeated contact with the lateral aspect of the greater trochanter from an external force. A fall directly on the side of the hip can contuse the bursa between the attachment of the gluteus medius and the greater trochanter.

SIGNS:

Pain and local tenderness over the greater trochanter are always present; at times a limp on the affected side will be present. Lying on the injured side on a hard surface produces pain.

TECHNIQUE:

Have the patient lie on the unaffected side with hips and knees flexed. Thin patients facilitate identification of the greater trochanter and the precise area of tenderness. Fill a 10-ml luer-lock syringe with 20 mg prednisolone in 1 percent lidocaine, and depending upon soft tissue thickness, fit to it a sharp 1.5-inch 25-gauge or 3-inch 19-gauge cannula. Paint the skin directly above the tender greater trochanter with povidone iodine and insert the cannula down to the bone. If injection gives a burning pain, the anaesthetic is entering the inflamed bursa. Inject the entire 10-ml suspension by multiple puncture of the bursa, using as few skin penetrations as possible.

Second Visit: If symptoms continue for more than five days, repeat the treatment a week later.

Effectiveness: Treatment within one week after onset of disability gives better results. Usually one visit is sufficient for lasting relief from pain. After a month of symptoms, several treatments, a week apart, will be required.

The Leg

"Shin Splints"
(Anterior Tibialis)

INJURY:
Partial tearing of the periosteum with hemorrhage along the medial aspect of the tibia results from pounding on a hard surface while running. Many road runners encounter this at the beginning of a new season.

SIGNS:
Usually present bilaterally. Pain on fast walking and especially on running is present along the medial tibial border. Local swelling with marked tenderness is often present. Resisted dorsiflexion will usually reproduce the pain.

TECHNIQUE:
Two methods of treatment are corticosteroids injected locally with lidocaine or 8 percent dextrose in lidocaine. Treat alternate legs a week apart. Patients often refuse to stop running and improvement is therefore slow. A sharp ⅝-inch 25-gauge cannula is employed to inject 1 percent lidocaine with 1 mg prednisolone per ml. Tenderness is relieved by injecting at intervals of 2 cm, using 0.2 ml on the surface of the periosteum. To avoid a pincushion effect, 1-ml injections layered on the periosteum at intervals of 10 cm can be tried. I prefer to use 8 percent dextrose in 1 percent lidocaine injected into the periosteum down to bone at 2-cm intervals doing one "shin" at a time. No running should be allowed.

Second Visit: Repeat injection on the alternate tibia at one-week intervals. This may be done with a limit of three in each "shin."

Effectiveness: Cooperation of the patient is important for this treatment to be effective.

Strain of Gastrocnemius Muscle

INJURY:

A partial tear of the muscle-tendon junction occurs most often in the medial half of the gastrocnemius muscle.

SIGNS:

Sudden pain, as if from a baseball striking the leg, a sensation of snapping fibers, and pain when rising on the toes with knees straight are the major symptoms. A moderate amount of swelling comes on later.

TECHNIQUE:

Have the patient supine on the examining table with flexed hip adducted and externally rotated. With the knee flexed, carefully palpate the gastrocnemius to find the location and extent of injury. Mark this with povidone iodine and inject very sparingly with 5 mg prednisolone in 5 ml lidocaine using a sharp 1.5-inch 25-gauge cannula. Begin the injection around the periphery using 0.2-ml increments injecting in circular pattern from a central skin puncture. Complete freedom from pain and tenderness should be reached. Prescribe an inch heel lift and advise no stress of the calf muscles.

Second Visit: In one week a repeat injection with a maximum of 2.5 mg prednisolone in 5 ml 4 percent dextrose 1 percent lidocaine.

Effectiveness: Usually two treatments are enough, but four to six weeks of minimal contraction of the muscle is necessary for complete healing.

The Spine

We are a nation so engrossed in physical fitness that musculo-skeletal injuries are now occurring in all age groups, including those sixty-five years and up. Spine injuries are related to anatomical structure and give typical symptoms, which we can interpret with the help of a simple instructional guide. By eliminating major injuries resulting from traffic accidents, we can keep the scope of this chapter within reasonable limits. Before going into the mechanics of injury, diagnosis, and treatment, we need to define some terms. Objective findings are those anybody can see, while subjective symptoms are felt only by the disabled person. Muscle spasm is an objective finding. The muscles on the injured side are tightened up, bulging, and feel hard as a board to an examiner. Pain and a tight, tied-up feeling are your symptoms. When you have muscle spasm, all of the muscle fibers are contracting. When you normally move with muscle action, some, but not all, fibers are working. Pain is subjective. You feel it when sensory nerves are stimulated far beyond the normal. A fold of skin pinched moderately is felt as a squeeze, but pinching the skin with enough force to damage it is felt as pain. Pain is a warning and must be heeded to prevent serious injury. Referred pain is also subjective, but is not felt at the point where the nerve is stimulated. Referred pain is felt at a distance from the cause. It is related to the fact that injury to deep structures cannot be precisely localized. You not only feel the pain where the tissues are damaged, you also feel pain in a skin area that gets its sensory nerves from the same level in the spinal cord. This is called the dermatome basis of referred pain. Look at the diagram of the dermatomes and you'll see how intense pain can spread through spinal nerve connections in the cord to radiate into the buttock, thigh, knee, leg, and foot.

323

Pins-and-needles sensation is different from referred pain. The former travels down a nerve coming from the spinal cord and ends in muscles and skin areas. The numbness and tingling is like an electrical shock along the nerve. It means that something is pressing on the nerve, and it feels like the sensation you get when you hit the "funny bone" (really the nerve) on the inner side of your elbow.

Weakness is a very important finding. Weak muscles are unable to contract all their fibers fully because some of the nerve supply has been destroyed. When only a few fibers contract, the muscle is not able to do the necessary physical work. If it is a hip muscle, you will limp. If it is an arm muscle, you won't be able to lift and carry with that arm. Nerve injury in the neck is often diagnosed by the area of skin numbness or referred pain. Eight pairs of cervical nerves exit from the neck to go to the head, ears, neck, shoulders, arms, and hands. Above and below each cervical vertebra is a canal of exit so that C-1 has the first cervical nerve above and the second cervical nerve below. Last is the eighth nerve below the seventh vertebral body. Herniated discs in the cervical region will give typical pain patterns and numbness. You can tell where the trouble is by looking at a chart for the corresponding nerve-root areas. Referred pain from the cervical ligaments is different. It is sore locally and also at a distance in accordance with the dermatome chart. Traction relieves pressure on a nerve root, but makes a ligament hurt more. Neck muscle injuries are usually accompanied by muscle spasm and loss of motion. Injection of a local anaesthetic will relieve the spasm long enough to help make a diagnosis. Usually the ligaments and muscles are injured where they attach to bone. Pressure on the precise spot will give temporary relief by tiring the nerve conduction. The rest of this chapter will give you an introduction to treatment.

Cervical Interspinous Ligament Sprains

INJURY:

An uncontrolled range of hyperflexion will partially tear the interspinous ligaments in the midportion or at the periosteal attachment to bone.

SIGNS:

In addition to the subjective complaint of posterior neck pain, the patient has varying degrees of limitation of neck and head flexion associated with muscle spasm. One or more areas of severe local tenderness of the spinous processes and ligaments will be present.

TECHNIQUE:

Limited and protected head and neck flexion is obtained by having the patient prone on the examining table with a pillow beneath the chest and the forehead resting on the padded table surface. First identify all points of localized tenderness in ligaments and spinous processes and mark them with povidone iodine. Fill a luer-lock syringe with 1.5 ml 8 percent dextrose in 1 percent lidocaine for each area of skin marked with iodine. Use a sharp 1.5-inch cannula of 25 gauge to penetrate the skin down to the ligament or its attachment to the spinous process and inject the dextrose-lidocaine. Puncture the periosteum at 8-mm intervals through the same skin entry by withdrawing the point of the cannula to the subcutaneous layer and redirecting the cannula at an angle to cover a 3-cm area. Pain will be produced only in an area of injury and will last for less than 30 seconds. Complete anaesthesia will be present in 3 minutes.

Second Visit: Examination and treatment may be repeated at intervals of one or two weeks until improvement is present. Most patients will need from two to six visits. Progressive exercises to improve the range of rotation are prescribed when adequate relief from pain has been achieved. The possibility that pain is present because of other ligament and soft-tissue injuries must be kept in mind if symptoms continue after completion of ligament treatment.

Effectiveness: Improvement can be anticipated in 90 percent of patients in whom pain is due solely to interspinous ligament injury. If freedom from pain is not accomplished, a search for other causes of neck pain is required. Coincident litigation is a negative factor in early recovery.

Thoracic Interspinous Ligament Sprains

INJURY:

An episode of thoracic hyperflexion with or without a coincident vertebral compression fracture will markedly stress the supraspinous and interspinous ligaments above and below the area of compression.

SIGNS:

A kyphos will occur in compression fractures with prominence of the spinous process of the compressed vertebra. Local percussion pain and tenderness will be marked. All stressed ligaments will be painful and tender on pressure in both hyperflexion and fracture.

TECHNIQUE:

With the patient prone on the examining table, identify the points of bone and ligament tenderness with one fingertip. Mark the spinous processes with a short transverse stripe of povidone iodine at each level and the ligaments with short vertical stripes of iodine. Fill a 10-ml luer-lock syringe with enough 8 percent dextrose in 1 percent lidocaine to inject each area with 1.5-ml solution. Use a sharp 1.5-inch 25-gauge cannula and begin by inserting the point vertically into the dorsal periosteum near the tip of a spinous process. Inject ligament periosteum junctions with increments of 0.2-ml solution at intervals of 8 mm by withdrawing the point to the subcutaneous layer and reinserting at different angles to cover as large a surface as can be reached through one skin puncture. Treat the ligament in the same manner and continue injecting tender areas until the patient has no local tenderness. (See Fig. 14.)

Second Visit: A few patients will become totally free of symptoms after a single visit. The majority will need from two to six treatments. Frequency of treatment will depend upon the length of the recovery phase after injection and varies from one to three weeks. About 50 percent will become free of symptoms if the anaesthetic mixture can reach all painful areas; 10 percent will be relatively unimproved; and varying degrees of improvement will take place in the remaining 40 percent. Success depends upon the injury's being limited to the treated areas. Coincident litigation usually has some negative effect on results.

Effectiveness: My longest "cures" are in the thoracic group. This may be due to the marked limitation of motion in this area.

Lumbosacral Interspinous Ligament Sprains

INJURY:

Most back injuries occur in the lumbosacral area, where an increased range of motion accompanied by strong muscle action can cause multiple injuries. Stress of the interspinous ligaments during flexion is the major cause of supraspinous and interspinous tears. Compression fractures of the vertebral bodies stress the ligaments above and below the level of injury by increasing the interspinous distance.

SIGNS:

Pain is localized at the level of ligament tear. When complete rupture has taken place, a distinct hollow is present in the interspinous area. Patients complain that sitting is the most uncomfortable position and that they have a feeling of weakness with total loss of ability to run. Point tenderness is specific and can continue in conjunction with chronic pain and fatigue for years. Passive flexion of both hips with knees pressed against the chest will be painful at the level of injury.

TECHNIQUE:

Treatment is easiest with the patient in the prone position. A pillow beneath the abdomen will flatten the lumbar lordotic curve and old, very obese individuals with breathing impairment can be treated lying on the side with hips and knees flexed. Mark each tender interspinous ligament with povidone iodine. Fill a 10-ml luer-lock syringe with 8 percent dextrose in 1 percent lidocaine and fit it with a 1.5-inch 25-gauge sharp cannula. Some obese patients will require a longer cannula and pose a hazard of injection deep to the superficial ligaments. Keep this in mind and first determine the distance of the skin surface to the dorsal tip of the spinous process in order to establish the safe depth of injection. Place thumb and index finger of one hand on each side of a spinous process to permit centering of the cannula and insert the sharp cannula through the skin at the midpoint of the ligament. Slowly inject about 1 ml solution while you are withdrawing the point from the deep layers toward the supraspinous ligament. A sharp exclamation from the patient will identify the injured supraspinous ligament. After the point reaches the subcutaneous layer, change the angle of injection to permit reaching the ligament's periosteal attachment to the spinous process and inject 0.2-ml increments of dextrose-lidocaine at 8-mm intervals until all pain is relieved. Treat each interval and allow several minutes for full anaesthetic effect before testing for residual pain by passively hyperflexing the lumbosacral spine. Complete relief from pain indicates a very good prognosis for an ultimate "cure." Failure to obtain complete relief indicates the presence of injury to structures in addition to the interspinous ligaments.

Second Visit: Repeat treatments may be given at intervals of one or two weeks, depending upon the degree of postinjection pain and its duration. Up to 5 percent of patients will need only one treatment visit; 50 percent will fail to improve. Varying degrees of improvement will be obtained in the remainder.

Effectiveness: Long-term "cure" will depend on the nature of healing in each patient. The stress that caused the original disability can, if repeated, reinjure the same tissues. Smoking more than one pack of cigarettes daily prevents adequate healing, as does extreme obesity. Some of my patients with a twenty-year follow-up are still free from pain.

Sacroiliac Ligament Sprains

INJURY:

Sprains of the sacroiliac ligaments are extremely common. Avulsion of portions of the sacroiliac ligament are also common. Injury to both joints can cause a range of slight to total disability in these patients.

SIGNS:

Pain is felt across the lower portion of the back on one side or both sides. Deep sacroiliac pain with radiation into the groin, thigh, or leg on the injured side may also be present. Percussion over the lateral ilium will reproduce the pain on the side of injury. A positive Trendelenburg limp and thigh-muscle atrophy are present in long-standing cases. Injection of the injured ligaments is painful, but complete relief from pain will occur within five minutes of injection and permit rapid diagnosis. Stress of the joint ligaments by manipulation and standing on the affected lower extremity will usually produce typical pain.

TECHNIQUE:

Patient prone is the preferred position, although obesity and pregnancy will require treatment with the patient lying on the side. Identify the bony prominence of both iliac crests down to the sacrum and sketch this outline on each side with povidone iodine. Mark the skin in the midline of the back at the level between L5 and S1. Fill a 10-ml luer-lock syringe with 8 percent dextrose in 1 percent lidocaine and attach a 3.5-inch 19-gauge short-bevel sharp cannula. Puncture the skin through the midline at an angle of 45° at the iodine mark. Insert the cannula diagonally through the lumbar muscles aiming at the proximal level of the sacroiliac joint until you reach iliac attachments of the sacroiliac ligaments. Inject 0.3 ml solution very slowly to avoid producing severe pain. Partially withdraw the point and direct it medially to inject the sacral attachment at the same level. Inject at intervals of 8 mm, moving distally along the margins of the joint into the ligamentous attachments. At first the patient will complain of severe pain during each injection, but complete relief from pain occurs within five minutes. Inject the distal superficial sacroiliac ligaments with a 25-gauge 1.5-inch sharp cannula adjacent to the inferior medial border of the posterior iliac crest. Limit the volume of dextrose-fortified anaesthetic to 1 ml of 1 percent lidocaine per ten pounds of body weight. Posttreatment pain is usually controlled by buffered aspirin or the more readily tolerated magnesium trisalicylate. (See Fig. 15.)

Second Visit: An occasional patient will have no symptoms when returning for follow-up care. Repeat treatments can be given at one- or two-week intervals. Repeat that portion of the first examination that was positive for sacroiliac injury before giving the second series of injections. Less pain and fewer points of severe pain will be found. A narrow sacroiliac belt binding the pelvis tightly will give symptomatic relief during the early phases of injection treatment.

Effectiveness: Complete freedom from pain and injection tenderness can be obtained after three to six visits.

Muscular Disabilities of the Lumbar Spine

INJURY:
Strain of muscle fibers from maximum contraction effort results in tearing of muscle fibers with local areas of necrosis and inflammation. Compression from local contusion gives a similar injury with more hemorrhage evident.

SIGNS:
Pain, tenderness, and often muscle spasm are present. Old untreated muscular injuries often have localized areas of scarring which are highly sensitive and act as trigger points for the production of acute pain or muscle spasm.

TECHNIQUE:
With the patient prone, examine the lumbar area and mark all points of tenderness with povidone iodine. Painful areas that contain nodular trigger points will need special treatment. Look for muscle spasm and atrophy. If three or more areas are to be treated, fill a 10-ml syringe with 20 mg prednisolone in 1 percent lidocaine and fit it with a sharp 1.5-inch 25-gauge cannula. Be sure to identify the hard nodule of a trigger point by the increased resistance to the penetration by the cannula and inject one or two ml. Treat larger areas by injecting with multiple diagonal penetrations from a single skin puncture.

Second Visit: Repeat the treatment after one week if pain is still present.

Effectiveness: Two treatments are usually adequate. If pain and disability continue, look for factors outside the muscle boundaries for the basic cause. A nerve root compression syndrome, ligament injuries, or injury to contiguous joints can affect the nearby muscles.

Muscular Disabilities of the Gluteal Area

INJURY:
Compression and stress injuries will partially tear muscle fibers and alter the patient's gait.

SIGNS:
Pain, tenderness, and often muscle spasm are present. Compression of the injured muscle may evoke referred pain down the thigh. Gluteus medius injuries demonstrate a limping gait and a positive Trendelenburg test with a lowering of the nonweight-bearing hip instead of elevation. Gluteus maximus injuries are characterized by a peculiar lurch, in which the patient leans backward with each step on the injured side.

TECHNIQUE:
With the patient prone, probe the gluteal muscles with a fingertip and mark the areas of acute tenderness with povidone iodine. Fill a 10-ml syringe with 20 mg prednisolone and 1 percent lidocaine. If painful nodules are present, inject them with 2 ml steroid suspension by multiple puncture. Identify the hard fibrous nodule by sensing the increased resistance to penetration by the sharp cannula. A 1.5-inch 25-gauge cannula is adequate for most patients. Use a single skin puncture to treat a 10-cm radius of muscle by partially withdrawing and redirecting the cannula during the injection.

Second Visit: Repeat the treatment in one week if disability is still present.

Effectiveness: Rapid improvement can occur after a single treatment. If pain is still present after the second treatment, look for causes outside the boundaries of the affected muscle. Nerve root and ligament injuries are suspect.

Index